TRANSFORMATIVE
PLANNING

ACHE Management Series

TRANSFORMATIVE
PLANNING

How Your Healthcare Organization Can Strategize for an Uncertain Future

JIM AUSTIN

ACHE Management Series

Your board, staff, or clients may also benefit from this book's insight. For information on quantity discounts, contact the Health Administration Press Marketing Manager at (312) 424-9450.

This publication is intended to provide accurate and authoritative information in regard to the subject matter covered. It is sold, or otherwise provided, with the understanding that the publisher is not engaged in rendering professional services. If professional advice or other expert assistance is required, the services of a competent professional should be sought.

The statements and opinions contained in this book are strictly those of the author and do not represent the official positions of the American College of Healthcare Executives or the Foundation of the American College of Healthcare Executives.

22 21   20   19   5   4   3   2

Library of Congress Cataloging-in-Publication Data
Names: Austin, Jim (Editor of Leading strategic change in an era of
   healthcare transformation), author.
Title: Transformative planning : how your healthcare organization can
   strategize for an uncertain future / Jim Austin.
Description: Chicago, IL : Health Administration Press, [2018] | Series:
   HAP/ACHE management series | Includes bibliographical references and
   index.
Identifiers: LCCN 2017057191 (print) | LCCN 2017055806 (ebook) | ISBN
   9781567939811 (ebook) | ISBN 9781567939828 (xml) | ISBN 9781567939835
   (epub) | ISBN 9781567939842 (mobi) | ISBN 9781567939804 (alk. paper)
Subjects: | MESH: Delivery of Health Care—organization & administration |
   Health Services Administration | Organizational Innovation | United States
Classification: LCC RA971 (print) | LCC RA971 (ebook) | NLM W 84 AA1 | DDC
   362.1068—dc23
LC record available at https://lccn.loc.gov/2017057191

The paper used in this publication meets the minimum requirements of American National Standard for Information Sciences—Permanence of Paper for Printed Library Materials, ANSI Z39.48-1984. ♾ ™

Acquisitions editor: Jennette McClain; Project manager: Joyce Dunne; Cover designer: Brad Norr; Layout: PerfecType

Found an error or a typo? We want to know! Please e-mail it to hapbooks@ache.org, mentioning the book's title and putting "Book Error" in the subject line.

For photocopying and copyright information, please contact Copyright Clearance Center at www.copyright.com or at (978) 750-8400.

Health Administration Press
A division of the Foundation of the American
   College of Healthcare Executives
300 S. Riverside Plaza, Suite 1900
Chicago, IL 60606-6698
(312) 424-2800

To my family, Susan, Tanner, and Sam, and to my dad, Dr. James Austin (1927–2017).

Contents

Preface

MY DAD WAS a physician. My earliest memories were of Sunday family meals in the hospital cafeteria, down the hill from our home, just outside Boston. It was my first experience with a restaurant offering unlimited choice—or so I thought until my parents informed me that I had to finish *everything* I put on my plate.

In a way, we are dealing with similar issues today. How much choice should we have in healthcare? What will each of us be responsible for? What is the balance between the private-market provision of services and public care? More fundamentally, is healthcare a right, or is it a service to be "earned" on the basis of income, need, insurance coverage, or some other measure?

While these are critical questions, they are not the focus of this book. Rather, this book is for those healthcare leadership teams across the healthcare spectrum struggling to define a strategic direction and execution plan given the range of uncertainties they face. In the military, the fog of battle is now characterized as a VUCA world: **v**olatile, **u**ncertain, **c**omplex, and **a**mbiguous—an apt characterization of the US healthcare system as well.

How, then, can leaders plan for, and ideally embrace, such uncertainties? This book is a how-to, strategic planning manual for healthcare leadership teams facing the ever more challenging VUCA world of US healthcare.

One theme found throughout the book is the need for healthcare leaders to consider transformative change, which is fundamentally different than incremental change. As John Kotter explains (Kotter and Cohen 2002, ix):

> By transform, I mean the adoption of new technologies, major strategic shifts, process reengineering, mergers and acquisitions, restructurings into different sorts of business units, attempts to significantly improve innovation, and cultural change.

Incremental change—improving current operations, raising quality metrics, enhancing patient satisfaction scores—is essential. But these efforts are not enough to meet the changing demands of the US healthcare system. Hospitals and health systems must also pursue transformative change to expand the way healthcare is managed, financed, and delivered.

This mandate raises three challenges for healthcare leaders. First, while incremental change may be insufficient, it is a necessary precondition for driving transformative developments. Only by freeing up resources from increasingly efficient operations can organizations invest in transformative initiatives, which typically take several years to yield positive returns. Hence the focus of this book: meeting the needs of today *and* tomorrow.

Second, while incremental changes to existing, ongoing operations can be identified through a review of past efforts, in times of uncertainty requiring more transformative responses, the past is *not* prologue, to contradict the expression "What's past is prologue" from Shakespeare's (2017) *The Tempest*. (For a more detailed discussion of transformative change, see Austin, Bentkover, and Chait 2016, 3–4.) The definition of true uncertainty—as opposed to risk management—is that the future will not be similar to the past, possibly not even in the realm of what was foundational in the past. True uncertainty means that no data set is readily available to define future choices. (Note that the term *uncertainty* as used in this book is not meant to describe so-called black swan events, or those that occur once in a hundred years. For an exploration of uncertainty in terms of rarely occurring events, see Taleb 2010.)

Third, truly transformational change transcends existing systems. Its effects are best realized when the past ways of operating are restructured, revised in ways that are difficult to envision on the basis of past perspectives. For example, electricity influenced manufacturing processes only when "factories themselves were reconfigured" (Harford 2017, 18) in the 1920s—not when electric motors replaced steam-driven motors in the late 1800s. More recently, companies that merely invested in computers in the late 1990s saw few immediate benefits, unlike those entities that reconfigured their operations, "decentralizing, outsourcing and customizing their products" (Harford 2017, 18), to realize enormous productivity gains.

Do these lessons mean that leadership teams have no strategic guidelines or teachings from the past that can inform future choices? No, and this book aims to guide leadership teams struggling with the following parallel demands:

- How to keep current operations going while layering on new or transformative initiatives so the organization can be successful no matter how the future evolves
- How to improve the execution of the new plans

Specifically, how should leadership teams plan for the range of uncertainties they face? To mention a few:

- Will payment in the future US healthcare system be based primarily on fee-for-service charges or on measures related to outcomes?
- Will hospitals maintain their current focus on treating the sick who appear at their doors, or will they shift to a population health approach whereby they seek to keep people *out* of the medical facility by elevating and maintaining the community's health status?

- Will greater emphasis be placed on local payment and care networks, with the federal government shifting responsibilities to states, for example, or will national payment and delivery systems (e.g., similar to Medicare) emerge? Consider that a number of states, such as Washington, Vermont, California, and Massachusetts, are in the process of pioneering new healthcare reimbursement and delivery systems, often starting with Medicare as the payment model (see, e.g., Washington State Health Care Authority 2017).

The premise of this book is that no one knows the answer to these critical questions. The actual predictive power of forecasters, especially the further out one looks, is no better than flipping a coin. For example, Tetlock and Gardner (2015) found that professional prognosticators often get locked into one point of view and thus are often bested by amateur forecasters with a "growth mind-set": balancing determination, self-reflection, and an openness to learning from one's mistakes. Thus, leadership teams need to embrace uncertainty—particularly for long institutional planning time frames—by implementing the following tools and processes:

1. Develop a **portfolio of options** that creates the capacity to respond in an agile way to future changes in the short and long term.
2. Drive **agreed-on changes**—incremental and transformational—throughout the organization that are based on clear, consistent answers to two questions: Why do we need to change, and who is responsible for effecting which changes?
3. Establish **environmental monitoring efforts** that alert leaders to trends sooner rather than later.

The four steps recommended in this book to implement these measures are summarized in exhibit P.1.

Exhibit P.1: Four-Step Process for Leading Transformational Change

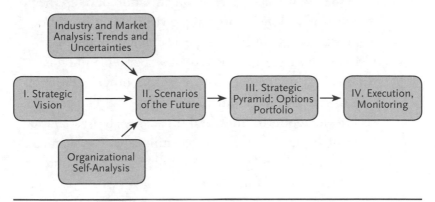

To describe this four-step process, this book is organized into the following chapters:

- *Chapter 1: Mental Models and Strategic Decision Making.* Any strategic planning effort is only as good as the decision-making processes that lead to strategic choices. This chapter, a precursor to describing the actual strategic planning process, outlines the four critical decision traps—frame bias, overconfidence, groupthink, and attribution bias—leadership teams must overcome to be open to new, transformative opportunities and challenges.

- *Chapter 2: Front and Back—Vision and the Strategic Pyramid.* Transformative strategy development begins with a vision that emotionally engages the organization. Any transformation starts by answering: Why change? The strategic planning effort concludes with a portfolio of strategic initiatives—the strategic pyramid—that both keeps the current organization operating ever more efficiently and expands into new, transformative efforts for sustainable competitive advantage.

- *Chapter 3: Strategy Development for a VUCA World—Scenario Planning.* In times of uncertainty, the past is not prologue. How, then, does an organization develop the portfolio of options for its unique vision as outlined in chapter 2? To expand the strategic dialogue and choices of the leadership team, the tool of scenario planning is explored in this chapter. Different from other traditional tools of strategy development, such as a SWOT (strengths, weaknesses, opportunities, and threats) analysis, scenario planning begins in the future, creating a reasonable range of potential futures by which to explore winning strategies no matter how the future evolves.
- *Chapter 4: Successful Execution.* A three-part framework defined by clarity, feasibility, and accountability is outlined to help leadership teams overcome the myriad reasons most strategic change efforts fail. In addition, given the ongoing uncertainties of the US healthcare environment, leadership teams must constantly monitor from the outside in, building flexibility into their plans.

The final choices any leadership team makes depend on the institution's vision, strategy, resources, and capabilities. This book was written to provide the essential frameworks and processes to guide such efforts, improving any team's chances of success in dealing with the challenging, evolving VUCA world of healthcare.

CHAPTER 1

Mental Models and Strategic Decision Making

*What gets us into trouble is not what we don't know.
It's what we know for sure that just ain't so.*

—Mark Twain

AT ITS HEART, strategy deals with an unknown future. Strategic planning should be the one opportunity to challenge past actions and assess a range of future investments to establish a path forward into the ever-evolving future. Thus, strategy should be a creative act. Unfortunately, most strategic planning efforts accomplish little more than incremental changes to past activities, even when faced with challenges that are radically different than those encountered in the past. A leadership team's failures of strategy are often *failures to anticipate a reality different than what the team is prepared or willing to see.* As Steve Lohr (2007) writes in an article profiling Microsoft, "One of the evolutionary laws of business is that success breeds failure; the tactics and habits of earlier triumphs so often leave companies—even the biggest, most profitable and most admired companies—unable to adapt."

Thus, before outlining the tools for transformational strategic planning and execution in times of uncertainty, leaders must determine what decision-making processes are essential to the effort.

Approaching strategic planning with an unconstrained mind-set is critical to identifying and prioritizing future opportunities. Without such a mind-set, the resulting plan tends to look to the past, incrementally moving the healthcare organization forward while lacking the creativity and insights to layer on transformational changes critical for future success.

Daniel Kahneman notes (Lewis 2016, 198):

> In making predictions and judgments under uncertainty, people . . . rely on a limited number of heuristics which sometimes yield reasonable judgments and sometimes lead to severe and systemic error.

The good news, Kahneman, Lovallo, and Sibony (2011) argue, is:

> Executives can't do much about their own biases. . . . But given the proper tools, they can recognize and neutralize those of their teams.

Most of the time, decisions are made intuitively, quickly, and subconsciously. After all, problem solving, or thinking analytically, takes energy and time. "Going with your gut instinct" is easier, especially if one has deep content knowledge in the area and has dealt with comparable problems multiple times in the past. However, for more complex issues with major consequences, "Sober reflection is indispensable . . . logic trumps intuition" (Dobelli 2013, 305). The difficulty lies in distinguishing between the two situations. While Kahneman, Lovallo, and Sibony (2011) are not sanguine about the ability of individuals to correct their own decision-making errors, they say:

> There is reason for hope . . . when we move from the individual to the collective, from the decision maker to the decision-making process, and from the executive to the organization.

Thus, before outlining the best methodologies or tools for strategy development and transformational change, teams should step back and ask the following questions:

- *What major issues is the team trying to resolve, and what assumptions and potential options about them can be discerned?* For example, if part of the leadership team thinks the way forward is to reduce operating costs while another group assumes only innovative investments in new delivery models will drive future success, consensus will be hard to achieve when establishing future priorities.
- *What data will be essential to make fact-based, objective decisions?* Whether consciously or subconsciously, most individuals seek data sources that support their *existing* points of view. Even the Internet, which holds the promise of unlimited information, "is contributing to the polarization of America, as people surround themselves with people who think like them and hesitate to say anything different" (Miller 2014).
- *How will the leadership team make choices that are built from all points of view?* Leaders should avoid defaulting to the way things have always been done or, worse, making decisions that primarily reflect a powerful minority who wield influence. As articulated by David M. Cote, executive chairman of Honeywell International (Bryant 2013, emphasis added):

> Your job as a leader is to be right *at the end of the meeting*, not at the beginning of the meeting. It's your job to flush out all the facts, all the opinions, and at the end make a good decision, because *you'll get measured on whether you made a good decision*, and not whether it was your idea from the beginning.

- *Is the leadership team willing to change course?*
  Contemplation of a world that is **v**olatile, **u**ncertain, **c**omplex, and **a**mbiguous—a VUCA world—includes recognition and acceptance that the future will be different—possibly radically different—from the world of today. However, once decisions are made, the psychological "stickiness" of sunk costs, or expenditures made to bring those decisions to fruition, leads most teams to resist changing direction, even when presented with data that challenge the efficacy of past decisions (Dobelli 2013, 13–15).

DECISION MAKING AND DECISION TRAPS

How might a team best address these questions? Many articles and books have been written offering a variety of approaches to improving decision making (e.g., Schoemaker 2002; Ariely 2008; Kahneman 2011; Thaler and Sunstein 2008; Dobelli 2013); however, most are in agreement about the importance of the following four steps suggested by Russo and Schoemaker (2001):

1. Understand the issue(s).
2. Gather relevant, impartial information.
3. Make a fact-based, objective decision.
4. Be willing to reassess that decision on the basis of changing conditions and the degree of progress made.

One impediment for most organizations is the fact that individuals—and, by implication, teams—are hardwired to fall into one or more of the following decision traps while executing each of these steps:

- Frame narrowness
- Confirmation bias

- Groupthink
- Attribution bias

Healthcare leaders and their teams must work to overcome these decision traps. For example, prior to embarking on strategy development, teams should make sure they have appropriate processes in place, and take the time to review those processes, for overcoming each type of trap, as discussed in the following paragraphs.

Frame Narrowness

Leaders tend to want and expect to reach a solution quickly. Too often, however, they fail to spend adequate time considering the exact problem that needs to be addressed and uncovering the team's assumptions about the related issues. Some observers attribute that tendency to cave dwellers' primordial need to decide quickly whether that movement in the bush is a man-eating lion or just the wind, speculating that humans today frame problems rapidly, intuitively, and almost effortlessly.

To compound this desire to make decisions quickly, individuals rarely make their assumptions explicit, leaving the others on the team to guess about potential agendas or preferences. Furthermore, the lack of time spent assessing the true problem at hand leads teams to address nonissues or revisit previously resolved—or abandoned—concerns.

To avoid frame narrowness, at the beginning of a transformational strategic planning effort, ask each participant on the leadership team to independently answer the following questions:

- Why was our institution or group successful in the past?
- What needs to be done in the future to maintain, or increase our chances for continued, success?
- Looking forward, what assumptions does each participant have about the overall strategic planning effort? For

example, if several members of the strategic planning team assume whatever changes are made to healthcare coverage in the United States will only minimally affect ongoing operations, while several others assume the opposite, participants will struggle to find common ground because of their (often subconscious) assumptions. Only in calling out those assumptions and encouraging awareness of each member's "frame" can teams search creatively for solutions.

For further insights on framing and frame narrowness, see Wedell-Wedellsborg (2017).

What Is the Problem?

As an exercise to enhance team members' awareness of frame narrowness, ask the group to discuss the essential issue at the core of each of the following two real-world problems:

- Residents in an older building complain that the elevator is terribly slow. Management, while sympathetic, is unwilling to invest the millions of dollars needed to install a new elevator system.
- In the 1980s, Delta Air Lines experienced a number of nonfatal but highly embarrassing errors, such as planes landing at the wrong airport, which were usually the fault of decisions made by Delta pilots.

As the discussion progresses, observe how individuals frame the problem, especially the tendency to immediately propose a solution. The key to avoiding frame narrowness is to postpone fixing the problem until enough time has been spent eliciting opinions on what the real problem is. For example, in the elevator scenario, is the issue one of elevator speed and aging equipment, or are the complaints caused by some other factor? Have the team list other possible issues, come to a consensus on the core problem, and only then discuss possible cures.

How was the real-world elevator problem addressed? The building owners placed mirrors in the elevator waiting area, and complaints about the "terribly slow" wait times dropped to near zero. The building's management determined that the residents simply needed to occupy themselves while passing the time: by looking at themselves.

In the case of Delta Air Lines, the core problem was not a technical or even strictly a personnel issue but rather a cultural one. Traditionally, the chief pilot was never challenged once he made a decision—even when others in the cockpit felt the chief was wrong. Once this problem was diagnosed as one of status and deference in a culture characterized by rigid hierarchy, Delta engaged all of its pilots in breaking down those cultural norms; within six months of sensitivity training, landing errors disappeared.

Confirmation Bias

Leaders tend to make choices on the basis of a few experiences. The problem with that approach, as Paul Schoemaker (2002, 225) writes, is that "We are too sure of our single view about the future, and we fail to consider alternative views sufficiently." As a result, changing beliefs is difficult, as challenges to existing orthodoxy are often dismissed as irrelevant. Furthermore, such challenges to existing beliefs are emotionally difficult to handle (Festinger 1957) and, according to more recent research, desirability bias, or the tendency to trust the information one wants to believe, may further inhibit objectivity (Tappin, van der Leer, and McKay 2017).

Closely related to confirmation bias is **overconfidence**, or the belief that one is more knowledgeable or capable than he or she is in reality. Individuals—and collectively, teams—are notoriously

Confirmation Bias/Overconfidence: The Financial Meltdown of 2007–2008—Did Anyone See It Coming?

"Even though annual housing prices had not declined in nominal terms in modern memory, the forecasts of continued market growth with containable downside risks made no sense to hedge fund analyst [Steve] Eisman. Mortgages had become too easy to obtain. He and a few colleagues dove into the data, collected input from multiple sources, and spotted inconsistencies in the performance of the housing market. They worked through the longer-term consequences and realized that none of the possible outcomes justified the market's increasing exuberance.

"Eisman's ability to spot ambiguous threats and opportunities at the periphery of his business is rare among leaders. For several years, he resisted the temptation to do what everybody else was doing: going for the quick buck. Instead, he shorted the subprime mortgage market, and his fortitude paid off: Eisman's wider scanning and earlier detection yielded around US$1.5 billion for his hedge fund, **FrontPoint Partners**, a subsidiary of **Morgan Stanley**. His actions exemplify what **Nate Silver** [in his book *The Signal and the Noise*] calls 'the Prediction Paradox'. The paradox is that, the more humility we have about our ability to make predictions, the more successful we can be at anticipation. Why? Because open-mindedness encourages inquiry, debate and doubt."

Source: Excerpted from Schoemaker and Krupp (2015); emphasis in original.

error prone when assessing the risks of a given situation objectively, such that they underestimate the extent to which risks will derail them or their efforts. Similarly, people tend to overestimate their abilities, as demonstrated in the following examples (Dobelli 2013, 44; Thaler and Sunstein 2008, 32):

- 93 percent of US student drivers think they are "above average" drivers.
- 68 percent of University of Nebraska professors rated themselves in the top 25 percent for teaching ability.
- Entrepreneurs starting new businesses say their chances for success are 90 percent—when statistics show a 50 percent failure rate on average.

While perhaps comical, these examples point to fundamental ways in which individuals are "predictably irrational": First, most leaders believe they have more control over their business and the external environment than they do. According to studies reviewed by Schoemaker (2002, 6), "While managers concentrate most of their energies on the existing business, the management of external uncertainty may have more potential for creating value." In fact, as shown in exhibit 1.1, nearly half of an entity's return on assets results from external influences over which executives have no control (Roquebert, Phillips, and Westfall 1996).

Second, as Yale University economist Robert Schiller explains, "people tend to make judgments in uncertain situations by looking for familiar patterns and *assuming future patterns will resemble past ones*, without sufficient consideration of the reasons for the pattern or the probability of the pattern repeating itself" (de Jong 2015, 124; emphasis added). Yet, in times of uncertainty, the past is *not* a guide to the future.

Before the leadership team begins to examine the strategic implications of healthcare reform and gather relevant data, it should discuss the following questions:

Exhibit 1.1: Drivers of Return on Managed Capital

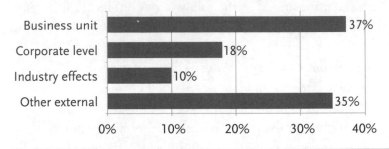

How much is the variance due to actions/influence from the . . .

Business unit	37%
Corporate level	18%
Industry effects	10%
Other external	35%

Source: Roquebert, Phillips, and Westfall (1996).
Note: Return on managed capital is profit realized relative to the amount invested.

- Where are we too reliant on a *single, common view of our strategic options*?
- Who can provide an *alternative perspective* on the data we will examine to help us broaden our strategic planning efforts and avoid strategic "myopia"?
- How can we avoid overconfidence through exploring a range of *perspectives* inside and outside of our group?

Groupthink

At a subconscious level, most individuals want to be part of a group, a member of the so-called A team. After all, the worst form of punishment is considered by many to be solitary confinement. Once an individual is part of a group, he or she has difficulty challenging the prevailing mores or beliefs of that group. Individuals quickly understand what is and is not acceptable in their team, such as what the boss or most senior person wants to hear and what topics of discussion are out of bounds (Asch 1955).

Even when teams are admonished to challenge existing ortho-doxies in brainstorming sessions, for example, team members often stifle their innermost thoughts to fit with prevailing team norms.

Janis and the Power of Groupthink

Irving Janis (1972), a leading academic in the study of *groupthink* (a term coined by William Whyte in 1952 in *Fortune* [Whyte 2012]), described it as (de Jong 2015, 137):

> the mode of thinking that persons engage in when concurrence-seeking becomes so dominant in a cohesive in-group that it tends to override realistic appraisal of alternative courses of action. The more amiability and *esprit de corps* there is among the members of the policy-making in-groups, the greater the danger that independent critical thinking will be replaced by groupthink, which is likely to result in irrational and dehumanizing actions directed against out-groups.

Specifically, Janis argued that groupthink is powerful because of the following factors:

- Members cultivate a team spirit, often fostered by a strong leader.
- Often (subconsciously), members feel superior to those outside the group.
- Contact with outsiders or nonteam members is limited.
- Little dissent is voiced to preserve team unanimity.
- Members are (emotionally) content to be part of the team.

Therefore, as Adam Grant (2016) explains, before beginning a group brainstorming effort, team leaders should require each person to generate his or her ideas individually and then come together to brainstorm. Grant (2016, 10) notes:

> For a culture of originality to flourish, employees must feel free to contribute their wildest ideas. But they are often afraid to speak up, even if they've never seen anything bad happen to those [who] do.

To assess transformational opportunities, groups must be willing to challenge existing orthodoxy—to break groupthink. Part of the problem with disrupting groupthink, however, is that groupthink can expand a team's capabilities. When resolving issues of high complexity, we must rely on the expertise of others. As Yuval Harari (2017, 15) writes:

> From an evolutionary perspective, trusting in the knowledge of others has worked extremely well for humans.

But when groups become echo chambers of like-minded colleagues, reliant on data that reinforce existing points of view and loyalties, Harari explains (2017, 15):

> Most of our views are shaped by communal groupthink rather than individual rationality, and we cling to those views because of group loyalty. Bombarding people with facts and exposing their individual ignorance is likely to backfire.

Two possible frameworks or approaches may help teams avoid the perils of groupthink. The first, proposed by Kathleen Eisenhardt, an anthropologist at Stanford University, and colleagues studying how Silicon Valley management teams made tough, strategic decisions, derives from the observation that best-in-class firms—the

JFK and the Cuban Missile Crisis

US President John F. Kennedy assembled a cabinet known as "the best and the brightest." Yet, as a group, they supported the Bay of Pigs invasion, a military operation to support insurgents against Cuba's communist leader Fidel Castro, resulting in a spectacular failure. Fourteen months later, Kennedy faced another major challenge, which became known as the Cuban Missile Crisis. The Soviet Union was in the process of supplying 20,000 ground troops and tactical atomic weapons to Cuba, an island just 90 miles from the southernmost point of the United States. Most historians credit Kennedy with skillfully handling the Cuban Missile Crisis, as, in a departure from the Bay of Pigs decision making, he overcame the cabinet's tendency to demonstrate groupthink. What changed? Russo and Schoemaker (2001) note that Kennedy

- created two separate working groups to develop options;
- stopped attending meetings, as even senior leaders were uncomfortable challenging the president;
- requested the options be presented to him, inviting outside advisers to comment; and
- designated two key advisers as critics to question him throughout the decision-making process.

Russo and Schoemaker (2001, 168) conclude, "After nearly two weeks of discussion, Kennedy ordered the island blockaded. Six days later Soviet prime minister [Nikita] Khrushchev agreed to remove the missiles."

best-performing companies across different industries—consistently apply the following four strategies in their management meetings (Eisenhardt, Kahwajy, and Bourgeois 1997):

- *Independent data.* They begin discussions by asking: "What *independent, third-party data* do we have that are relevant for this issue(s)?" Rarely do they rely on in-house sources of information. If such independent, third-party data are not available or are insufficient, they stopped discussions until they could obtain such information. In those cases where a decision is required immediately and third-party data are not available, these teams make the best decision possible on the basis of available evidence, subject to review once independent data can be found or generated, thereby offsetting confirmation bias.
- *Brainstorming as part of the decision-making process.* With the independent data in hand, high-performing teams list any and all options that emerge from a brainstorming session. No potential solution or explanation is rejected. Rather, the effort is focused on understanding what the situation requires from as many angles as possible, thus offsetting frame narrowness.
- *Clear decision rules.* At the end of the brainstorming portion of the meeting, a designated individual or a small executive team makes the decision. Those decision rights are agreed on prior to the meeting. Eisenhardt, Kahwajy, and Bourgeois (1997) found that as long as all the participants feel their ideas are fairly presented and given consideration by the decision maker(s), team members demonstrate a high level of support for decisions, a threshold that is critical for execution to be effective (see chapter 4).
- *Trust.* Team members at best-in-class firms trust and like each other. The challenge with such a high level of affinity is in balancing the need for diversity of viewpoints with cultivating trust. If teams constitute themselves on the basis of "those we like," they may end up lacking diversity of perspective, which is essential in dealing with uncertainty and change (Grant 2016).

The second approach, instituted by Kleiner Perkins Caufield & Byers (KPCB)—one of the most successful US venture capital firms in history—is called the *balance sheet process*, and it is used to bring forth different points of view (see exhibit 1.2).

When the firm faces a major strategic decision—whether to raise a new fund, change its investing criteria, or shuffle the leadership at an acquired firm, for example—each partner completes the balance sheet from his or her point of view to indicate the pluses and minuses of the proposed action. A first critical step in the process is that, before they come together to discuss the proposal, each partner provides the others with background documents (notes detailing the individuals' ideas, rationales, and other considerations in preparing the balance sheet) ahead of time so that each partner can prepare his or her individual response. Second, before decision making begins, they go around the meeting room and read from their balance sheets. By being "forced to listen to the views of others first," partners at KPCB report they have changed their original points of view (Lovallo and Sibony 2010). The essential element of this exercise is to *delay* discussion, as the moment discussion begins, listening stops or becomes difficult because of the human penchant to shift from "taking in" to "pushing out"—to stop listening in the rush to explain one's own ideas or point of view (Kahneman 2011).

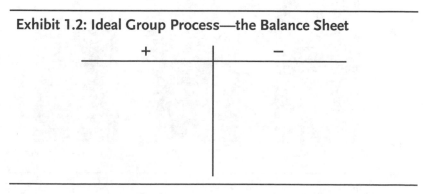

Exhibit 1.2: Ideal Group Process—the Balance Sheet

+	−

Source: Lovallo and Sibony (2010).

Attribution Bias

Objectively speaking, how are causes identified and attributed once decisions are made and outcomes realized? To ask the question differently, how easy is it to change course when new data are presented? According to a study by Sull, Homkes, and Sull (2015) on why execution fails, most organizations report that moving people or resources when markets change is extremely difficult (see exhibit 1.3).

Humans tend to see failure as a reflection of one's personal abilities rather than as a potential outcome of the business effort that, even in failure, offers learning possibilities. Every leader has experienced less-than-optimal outcomes. The ability to learn from these challenges is one key differentiator between highly successful leaders and average performers (Bennis and Thomas 2002). Nonetheless, most people fear the downside of a proposed action *two to three times as much* as they welcome the upside (Kahneman 2011). Objectivity is often lacking when assessing progress toward meeting goals and determining what needs to be done to improve outcomes. When

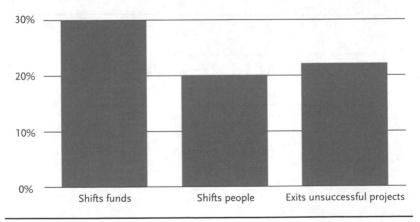

Exhibit 1.3: Rates of Adaptation to Changing Market Conditions
Percentage of senior executives who say their organization effectively . . .

Source: Sull, Homkes, and Sull (2015).

an individual or a team is successful, the individuals tend to laud personal efforts; when things do not go so well, team members often attribute the failure to external factors—pressures or issues that "no one could control." Examples of this tendency can be found in a study of quarterly reports released by Fortune 500 companies (Salancik and Meindl 1984):

- When budgets met the actual results, 79 percent of the performance was attributed to internal factors, thereby implying that what managers did was critical to success.
- In quarters that missed estimates, 75 percent of the blame was attributed to external factors.

Apart from individual responses to changing circumstances, healthcare's unique environment can also impede change. As Tucker and Edmondson (2003, 63) found in studying organizational failures at major hospitals:

The lack of organizational learning from failures can be explained instead by three less obvious, even counterintuitive, reasons: an emphasis on individual vigilance in health care, unit efficiency concerns, and empowerment (or a widely shared goal of developing units that can function without direct managerial assistance). These three factors, while seemingly beneficial for nurses and patients alike, can ironically leave nurses under-supported and overwhelmed in a system bound to have breakdowns because of the need to provide individualized treatments for patients.

In summary, as Warren Buffett states (Dobelli 2013, 19):

What the human being is best at doing is interpreting all new information so that their prior conclusions remain intact.

The challenge for leadership teams in facing the VUCA world of US healthcare is to be as objective as possible in seeking future opportunities—by understanding and preparing for how we are all predictably irrational. In his book *How Doctors Think*, Jerome Groopman, MD, writes that even when he has made a diagnosis, he tries to keep an open mind toward seeking other options (Groopman 2007, 66):

> Most errors are mistakes in our thinking. I learned from this to always hold back, to make sure that even when I think I have the answer, to generate a short list of alternatives . . . this simple strategy is one of the strongest safeguards against cognitive errors.

Generating that "short list of alternatives" is the focus of chapters 2 and 3.

CONCLUSION AND QUESTIONS HEALTHCARE LEADERS AND TEAMS SHOULD ASK

As Dan Ariely (2008) explains, individuals—and, consequently, the teams on which they participate—are predictably irrational in certain situations. The challenge is to be aware of the decision traps discussed in this chapter and build mechanisms into the strategic planning effort to mitigate potential shortcomings inherent in them (Kahnemann, Lovallo, and Sibony 2011). Therefore, before beginning the strategic planning effort itself (see chapter 2), the leadership team needs to assess *how* it will achieve the unconstrained, creative mind-set among team members that is critical for a robust strategic plan.

Questions

Specifically, leadership teams should discuss the following questions for each type of decision trap:

1. Framing/assumptions
   a. Why was the institution successful in the past?
   b. What needs to be done to be successful in the future?
   c. What could disrupt these ideas or perspectives?
2. Confirmation bias/overconfidence
   a. Is the leadership team relying on an overly narrow, shared view of the future?
   b. How can the leadership team gain fresh insights to broaden its strategic planning assumptions and perspectives?
   c. What can be done to leverage viewpoints inside and outside of the institution or group to challenge the tendency to focus on data that confirm existing beliefs?
3. Groupthink
   a. How will prevailing beliefs be challenged?
   b. Are all the points of view in the leadership team being surfaced and heard?
   c. What are the steps to reaching consensus? What will be the decision-making process?
4. Attribution bias
   a. What are the success metrics in broad terms for the strategic planning effort?
   b. How will progress to date be assessed, and how will the need to shift investments, people, and resources be triggered if circumstances change?
   c. How will the leadership team avoid the sunk-costs syndrome of spending more and more resources on losing strategic initiatives?

Front and Back—Vision and the Strategic Pyramid

Start with the end in mind.

—Stephen Covey

NOT ONLY SHOULD healthcare leaders take Covey's advice above and be clear on the end goal before beginning any effort, but they should begin "at the beginning," as the popular saying goes. In a changing, uncertain environment—the volatile, uncertain, complex, and ambiguous, or VUCA, world of US healthcare—leaders should create a flexible portfolio of initiatives that can both maintain current operations and layer on new capabilities to embrace the future. Leadership teams need to balance ongoing operational necessities with longer-term transformative initiatives, enabling their institutions to shift as external environments change.

This portfolio of initiatives—covering the short term, medium term, and long term with ever increasing levels of risk as well as reward—is the critical output or end of a flexible strategic planning effort (which then flows to execution; see chapter 4). But at the front end of transformative change, emotionally engaging all levels of the organization, resides the organizational vision (see exhibit 2.1).

For purposes of simplification, this book does not differentiate between a vision and a mission. Often, the former is viewed as the set of long-term, aspirational goals that are never accomplished, whereas a mission is seen as a short-term "call to action." As developed in chapters 3 and 4, the strategic portfolio constitutes the realization of that call to action, with a set of priorities that links strategy to execution.

DEVELOPING A VISION

Vision statements are important to organizational strategic planning for setting the following intentions:

- Aspirational goals that are rarely achieved but that serve as unwavering descriptors of an organization's "true north."
- A description of the organization's core purpose, or the rationale for its existence. As environments change, this sense of purpose may evolve.
- A broad sense of the scope and key capabilities that define the general positioning of the organization going forward.
- A unique statement to all employees of the emotional reasons for belonging to the institution's team.

Exhibit 2.1: Four-Step Process: Vision and Priorities

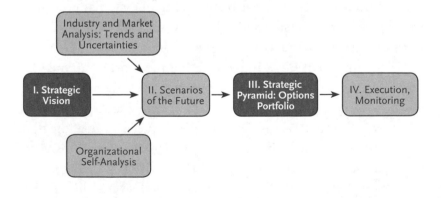

Some entities try to be "all things to all people." They fail to engage in the work of creating unique value, built on strategic differentiation and capabilities. For example, the following was, until recently, a large pharmaceutical company's vision statement:

> [The organization] will strive to achieve and sustain its leading place as the world's premier research-based pharmaceutical company. The company's continuing success benefits patients, customers, shareholders, business partners, families and the communities in which they operate all around the world. [Our] mission is to become the world's most valued company to all of these people.

This is pabulum; it is not emotionally uplifting, it certainly is not unique, and it is not aspirational (except possibly to shareholders). Compare that statement to a key component of Sony Corporation's vision (Collins and Porras 1996, 12):

> Become the company most known for changing the world-wide poor-quality image of Japanese products.

Sony's statement was formulated when the company was a small repair shop established shortly after World War II. Today, it remains part of the company's larger vision, a testament to Sony's enduring culture of quality.

Now consider Henry Ford's vision for the Model T automobile (Collins and Porras 1996, 10):

> I will build a car for the great multitude. It will be so low in price that no man making a good salary will be unable to own one—and enjoy with his family the blessing of hours of pleasure in God's great open spaces. . . . When I'm through everybody will be able to afford one, and everyone will have one. The horse will have disappeared from our highways.

Henry Ford was not selling an automobile; he was opening up the promise of America, enabling all to share in the country's bounty.

Vision statements get at why an organization exists—what is unique about its place in the market or business environment and what would be lost if it disappeared. Transformative change often

The Power of "Why"

In the late 1970s, Harvard University psychologist Ellen Langer instructed her research assistants to purposely "cut" in front of people waiting in line at the photocopiers in the library. The reason: to test the impact of "why." The researchers were to approach someone standing in line to make a copy, cut in front of that person, and utter one of the following three questions:

- *Version 1 (request only)*: "Excuse me, I have 5 pages. May I use the Xerox machine?"
- *Version 2 (request with a valid reason)*: "Excuse me, I have 5 pages. May I use the Xerox machine, because I'm in a rush and late for class?"
- *Version 3 (request with a fake or nonsensical reason)*: "Excuse me, I have 5 pages. May I use the Xerox machine, because I have to make copies?"

When the researchers analyzed the data, they found the following:

- In response to version 1, 60 percent of people let the researcher cut to the front of the line.
- For version 2, 94 percent of people let the researcher ahead in line.
- For version 3, 93 percent of people let the researcher ahead in line.

Langer's research became famous because it revealed one of the most powerful notions driving behavior: why. As long as we can justify behaviors ("I'm doing this because . . ."), we are more likely to continue with certain actions *even if the rationale makes little sense in the short term.*

Robert Cialdini (2006, 4), in his book *Influence*, writes, "A well-known principle of human behavior says that when we ask someone to do us a favor we will be more successful if we provide a reason. People simply like to have reasons for what they do" or, in this case, what they allow.

Source: Excerpted and adapted from Clear (2017).

starts when stakeholders sense a gap between the current direction of operations and what the organization should stand for or its core purpose. For example, is the overall vision of US healthcare providers primarily the delivery of a set of acute interventions by highly skilled, dedicated professionals? Or a more holistic aim of keeping the community healthy? One challenge facing many healthcare institutions today is the presence of a competing or unclear vision of the value and purpose of their place in the healthcare system.

Every year, on the last day of his lectures at Harvard Business School, Clayton Christensen (2010, 4) asks his students to reflect on three questions:

First, how can I be sure that I'll be happy in my career? Second, how can I be sure that my relationships with my spouse and my family become an enduring source of happiness? Third, how can I be sure I'll stay out of jail?

He argues that people do not start a career thinking they will look back feeling they wasted their time. No one gets married believing they will be divorced, and no one joins a company (such as Enron) assuming they will end up in jail. But individuals make

Core Purpose Examples

3M:

"To solve unsolved problems innovatively" (Collins and Porras 1996, 6)

Apple:

"We're on the face of the earth to make great products" (BehindTheHustle.com 2017)

Boeing:

"To push the leading edge of aviation, taking on huge challenges and doing what others cannot do" (Collins 2001, 5)

HP Development Company (formerly known as Hewlett-Packard):

"To make technical contributions for the advancement and welfare of humanity" (Collins and Porras 1996, 6)

Mary Kay:

"To give unlimited opportunity to women" (Collins and Porras 1996, 6)

Mayo Clinic:

"To provide the best care to every patient through integrated clinical practice, education and research" (Herzlinger, Huckman, and Lesser 2014, 2)

McKinsey & Company:

"To help leading corporations and governments be more successful" (Collins and Porras 1996, 6)

Merck:

"To preserve and improve human life" (Collins and Porras 1996, 6)

Nike:

"To experience the emotion of competition, winning, and crushing competitors" (Collins and Porras 1996, 6)

> Sony:
>
> > "To experience the joy of advancing and applying technology for the benefit of the public" (Collins and Porras 1996, 6)
>
> Wal-Mart:
>
> > "To give ordinary folk the chance to buy the same things as rich people" (Collins and Porras 1996, 6)
>
> Walt Disney Company:
>
> > "To make people happy" (Collins and Porras 1996, 6)

one short-term decision, then another short-term decision, and another short-term decision, and so on, only to find themselves a long way away from their true north. The need to calibrate—to match short-term choices against long-term, aspirational goals and values—underlies the importance of a vision.

How does a leadership team develop a worthy vision? First, it should not worry about wordsmithing. Inevitably, someone on the team argues about employing "and" versus "or" in a sentence, or some similar issue. While correct English is important, a vision stands or falls on its ideas. Specifically, a compelling vision has three components:

1. *An aspirational goal(s).* What organizational aims are considered slightly beyond reach? Just as important, how can these aims be described in vivid terms (similar to the earlier Henry Ford example)?
2. *A core purpose.* Why does the institution exist? A valuable exercise for the leadership team is to answer the question: "What would the world lose if our organization did not exist?" or "What value do we provide to internal and external stakeholders? To society?" Do not stop with the first set of responses. Asking the question(s) four

or five times consecutively typically reveals increasingly foundational levels of organizational purpose. In the context of the Toyota Production System and its related management training, such analyses are akin to the so-called five whys technique used to ascertain the root causes of performance issues.

3. *A set of stated values.* What are the organization's values, those cultural signposts that would be supported even if it hurt—even if to do so placed the entity at a competitive disadvantage? What does the organization stand for 100 years into the future, no matter what changes occur in the outside world? Furthermore, if a member of the organization does not share these values, or consistently undermines them, is such an individual—no matter how powerful—clearly unwelcome to remain in the organization? Many corporate values statements describe the same generic categories of honesty, integrity, sustainability, and so on without upholding them (Kunen 2002):

> [M]aybe adherence to ethical conduct really should go without saying. Every company's statement ends up rehashing the same things, anyway: We will maintain the highest ethical standards, treat our employees with respect. . . . As opposed to what? We will maintain fair-to-middling ethical standards?

A recent example indicative of the importance of values to corporate perception is the controversy over ride-sharing company Uber's alleged sexist culture. At Uber, the values include "always be hustlin'." By comparison, the stated values of competitor Lyft include "be yourself, uplift others, create fearlessly and participate" (Hook 2017, 20). A values statement should give employees guidance in choosing among alternatives. That means identifying a few high-priority values. In a study of heart attack outcomes across multiple hospitals, those institutions with the lowest readmission rates and highest returns on assets (Grant 2016, 93):

> spelled out no more than four organizational values. The more values [organizations] emphasized beyond that, the greater the odds that people interpreted them differently or didn't focus on the same ones.

One approach to putting the three essential components together is to create a narrative that follows the framework provided in exhibit 2.2.

An example of how these parts might come together for the vision of a subspecialty group is shown in exhibit 2.3.

Participants in Creating the Vision

Who should be involved in developing the organizational vision: the leadership team only, or a broader group of internal and external stakeholders? In times of radical or transformative change, a small group may be best positioned to develop, at the least, the main themes of the vision that can be discussed and refined by the broader

---

Exhibit 2.2: Creating a Vision Statement

"The . . . "	→	• Who are you? How are you identified?
"is . . . "	→	• What are you? What is the nature of your group?
"that . . . "	→	• What do you do? What products or services do you offer?
"for . . . "	→	• Whom do you serve? Are your clients /customers internal, external, or both?
"to . . . "	→	• Why do you exist? What value do you bring to your clients/customers? How do you support their mission?

Exhibit 2.3: Example of a Vision for a Clinical Subspecialty

The	*Orthopedics group*
is	*a collegial group of medical professionals from a broad variety of backgrounds*
that	*improves the lives of all we serve*
for	*our current and potential patients and communities*
to	*help individuals regain mobility and health and to reduce their pain no matter their ability to pay.*

organization. By engaging multiple levels of staff and management in refining and explaining the vision, a sense of ownership—an emotional connection—may be engendered. While finalizing the vision in this decentralized approach takes more time than a unilateral method does, less time may be required to drive commitment and action at all levels.

Should establishing or revising the vision be the first order of business for the leadership team's strategic planning efforts? Yes and no. It should be if the strategic plan builds on past efforts and the organization seeks primarily incremental change. However, if the entity faces pressure to implement transformative change, the leadership team should assess future environments and scenarios at the outset, and then swing back to develop the vision for the organization going forward. For example, in shifting from a fee-for-service business model to one embracing population health, the aspirational goals are dramatically different. Just how dramatic the change is may only be apparent after the leadership team has considered alternative future scenarios (this process is outlined in chapter 3).

In summary, a vision motivates and guides transformative change. It is the enduring true north that organizations can rally around in times of upheaval and uncertainty. In the words of Collins and Porras (1996, 2):

> Companies that enjoy enduring success have core values and a core purpose that remain fixed while their business strategies and practices endlessly adapt to a changing world.

THE STRATEGIC PYRAMID

The desired output of strategic planning efforts is a pyramid framework consisting of three types of initiatives: *core*, *new*, and *wow*. As presented here, the strategic pyramid is based on McKinsey & Company's "three horizons for growth" concept (Coley 2009) and is similar to Vijay Govindarajan's (2016) "box 1/box 2/box 3" framework.

The core, new, and wow elements and their interrelationships are shown in exhibit 2.4 and explained in the paragraphs that follow.

Exhibit 2.4: The Strategic Pyramid

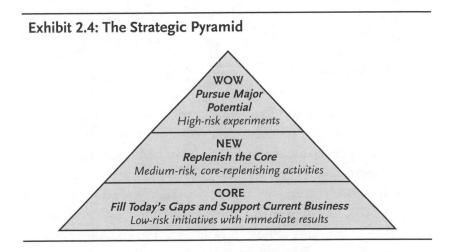

Core Initiatives

Core initiatives keep current operations running. These are the short-term, immediate activities that enable an institution or a group to meet its short-term commitments. Improved operating efficiencies are the focus for these efforts, thereby not only meeting current budgets and expectations but also freeing up resources for investments in future growth areas (new and wow). This aspect is critical because new and wow initiatives by definition do not add margin in the short term. For example, core initiatives could be quality and operational investments essential for meeting immediate budgetary, payer, and patient requirements. Virginia Mason Health System in Seattle calls these problems "rocks in your shoes"—the ongoing aggravations that challenge frontline managers' performance in times of change (Mate and Rakover 2016). As determined by examples from different industries, core strategic priorities represent 70 to 80 percent of the initiatives that existing institutions should focus on. Percentages are at best indicative of the state of the industry subsector and the lifecycle of the organization. For example, a start-up company may have a low percentage of core strategic initiatives; conversely, a mature business operating in a stable environment may have relatively few wow initiatives.

New Initiatives

Initiatives that are considered new in the context of the strategic pyramid are medium-term, moderate-risk priorities that over time can replenish or expand the core. They also might be current efforts that an organization eliminates or reduces to redirect resources to more important core or new growth activities (Viguerie, Smit, and Baghai 2008). Forming an accountable care organization or developing a risk-sharing relationship with several payers might be new strategic priorities. Typically, organizations target 10 to 20 percent of their resources or capabilities for new initiatives.

Wow Initiatives

Wow projects are those few experiments, or "pre–pre-feasibility" studies, that if successful may be pursued, opening up transformative growth opportunities. Note, however, that most of these initiatives are never realized. These are classic investment options whose guiding mantra should be: "Fail fast, fail cheap, and fail often." While potentially seductive, beware of focusing more than 5 to 10 percent of resources and management time on the ideas in this group.

Examples of wow initiatives might be changing the delivery model to a provider-sponsored health plan; adopting new social media platforms for reaching younger patients; or launching a medical tourism program using a few high-quality, non-US-based providers.

Indicative of the high-risk nature of initiatives in the wow category, several high-profile health plans (e.g., Catholic Health Initiatives, Piedmont Healthcare, Tenet Healthcare) recently exited the health insurance business (see, e.g., Evans 2016).

The goal of any strategy, as defined by Michael Porter (1996), is to achieve "sustainable competitive advantage." For not-for-profit organizations, some writers on strategy topics, such as Laurence Chait, prefer the term *sustainable competitive impact* (Austin, Bentkover,

---

Mayo Clinic's 2020 Strategic Plan: A Portfolio of Short-, Medium-, and Long-Term Initiatives

As discussed by Herzlinger, Huckman, and Lesser (2014), "The deliberations of the 2020 Initiative's steering committee, chaired by [John H. Noseworthy, MD] before he became [Mayo Clinic's] CEO, produced three strategic options for Mayo Clinic: (1) invest significantly to strengthen Mayo's traditional focus on tertiary and quaternary care; (2) maintain the Clinic's 'status quo' strategy while awaiting greater clarity around the changes

(continued)

(continued from previous page)

occasioned by the [Affordable Care Act]; and (3) aggressively pursue growth through alternative business models that would establish lasting relationships with patients and consumers as a complement to Mayo's existing tertiary and quaternary services. Facing limited capital and concerns about overcommitting the organization, the steering committee recommended the third option to the Board of Trustees."

What evolved was a tripartite strategic focus to achieve 200 million "customer touches" by 2020, defined as "giving the consumer what they want, when and where they want it, and on their terms" (Herzlinger, Huckman, and Lesser 2014). The strategic plan articulated a portfolio of initiatives organized by the following three areas:

- Run (i.e., continue to operate existing activities as efficiently and effectively as possible)
- Grow (i.e., expand current activities)
- Transform (i.e., pursue new products and business models)

Herzlinger, Huckman, and Lesser (2014) continue: "Several Mayo executives noted that the growth strategy required a greater appetite for risk-taking than that historically observed at Mayo Clinic. [David] Herbert [the executive responsible for developing new business models] said: 'If you take undue risks in the medical setting people may get hurt or die. So the risk appetite here, especially relative to the need for capital and growth, can be especially challenging. Operating at the speed of the marketplace, in my opinion, requires an ability to manage risk. I think we are managing it, but it has required a transition. It's not an area where [Mayo has] deep experience.'"

and Chait 2016, 25). While Porter's approach sounds reasonable, in reality it is almost impossible to realize. Rita Gunther McGrath (2012, 3), a professor at Columbia Business School at Columbia University and a leading authority on strategic thinking, writes:

> Few companies manage to prosper over the long term. Those that do are both more stable and more innovative than their competition.

In her study of nearly 4,800 publicly traded large companies (those with a market capitalization greater than $1 billion) over five years, and of just under 2,400 entities over a ten-year period, *less than 10 percent of those firms grew 5 percent every year*—slightly less than the annual global gross domestic product growth during her study period. How did these few outliers outperform their peers? Exhibit 2.5 summarizes McGrath's findings.

Exhibit 2.5: Practices of McGrath's "Outliers" for Sustaining Growth

- **Rapid adaptors:**
  - Make small bets and diversify their portfolios
  - Are active acquirers
  - Create processes that build flexibility
  - Build innovation into their processes

- **Champions of stability:**
  - Promote from within
  - Focus management on culture and shared values
  - Hold onto talent
  - Do not make radical strategy or portfolio shifts
  - Maintain a reliable customer base

Source: McGrath (2012).

Rationale for the Strategic Pyramid

Why is a portfolio of options—the strategic pyramid—the desired strategic planning output when facing a VUCA world? First, as McGrath (2012) identified, entities that succeed over time must both support their core and layer on transformative capabilities or activities to meet changing markets—the new and wow initiatives. The main issue is determining how to manage the balance among core, new, and wow initiatives, especially in challenging times.

Second, the strategic pyramid helps an organization focus on a few high-impact areas. As the example provided by DuPont indicates, at the most senior level of the several-billion-dollar division highlighted in exhibit 2.6, the leadership team concentrated on only nine projects.

Among the vast number of projects ongoing in a large division, the DuPont team identified only those few projects that could "make or break" its strategic plan. As one moves down the levels of the strategic pyramid, one sees how the supporting activities are created,

Exhibit 2.6: Prioritization of Initiatives at DuPont

Core	New	Experimental
Near Term/ Low Risk	**Medium Term/ Medium Risk**	**Long Term/ High Risk**
1. Project A	1. Project E	1. Project G
2. Project B	2. Project F	2. Project H
3. Project C		3. Project I
4. Project D		

DUPONT ®

Strengthen/extend core
Diversification
Leapfrog

• Prioritize projects within each category, comparing projects only within the same bucket.

Source: Adapted from the Product Development Institute, DuPont.

which serves to drive alignment throughout the organization. This is the third rationale for developing a strategic pyramid: It is the critical link between strategy and execution, which is explored further in chapter 4.

In developing its strategic plan, the leadership team should ideally create a list of major core, new, and wow investment priorities and then, on the bases of resources and capabilities, indicate those priorities to be acted on in the plan as well as those projects to be held in reserve (see exhibit 2.7).

If project A in the wow category fails to perform as desired, project B takes its place on the strategic plan. If someone comes up with a new idea or initiative after the strategic plan is approved, the project is placed in the relevant category and assessed against current efforts, establishing the new initiative's prioritization relative to those already on the list.

In this way, the strategic pyramid is the critical link between strategies and execution. Many strategic investments fail—not for being poorly formulated or for lacking in feasibility, but *because*

Exhibit 2.7: Ranking Strategic Initiatives

Core		New
X		1
XY		2
XW		3
SD		4
SX		
SS	**Wow**	
	A	
	B	
	C	

they are not executed. According to Jørgensen, Owen, and Neus (2008, 10), only 41 percent of strategic initiatives "fully met their objectives" (see exhibit 2.8).

Groups or organizations are unable to execute their strategic plans when they take on too many projects or do not establish clear accountabilities for carrying out strategic initiatives. Through the strategic pyramid framework, an individual or a team should be assigned responsibility for each of the major priorities articulated in the plan. On a regular basis, the leadership team reviews progress toward fulfilling the plan, calling on the relevant individual or team for an update (explored further in chapter 4).

Several other points related to the application of the strategic pyramid need to be considered as well, including the following issues:

- *What is a reasonable time frame?* It depends. In the midst of the 2007–2008 stock market meltdown, one financial

Exhibit 2.8: Success in Meeting Strategic Objectives

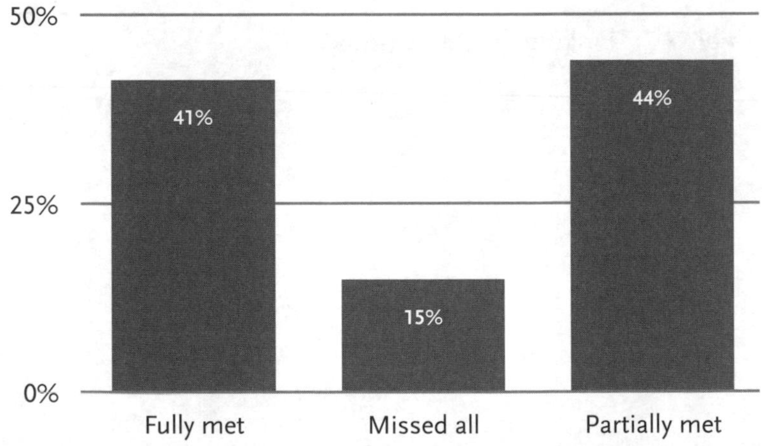

Source: Adapted from Jørgensen, Owen, and Neus (2008,10).

adviser stated in a Wharton Executive Education seminar, "My long-term plan is to survive 90 days." Conversely, for hospital capital projects that can take five to seven years from plan to completion, short term might be the normal planning cycle, while longer term could be ten or more years into the future. However, in most situations and for relatively mature organizations the following guidelines apply:

- Short term is typically the next 12 to 24 months.
- Medium term is often two to four years.
- Long term is considered more than four years.

- *How are projects prioritized?* Core and new ideas should be prioritized primarily via financial assessments such as net present value or return on investment (ROI) analyses. Do not use financial tools to prioritize ideas in the wow category, as these are experiments with little concrete knowledge available of their financial impacts. As Roch Parayre recommended in a communication with the author, "Use ROI—meaning return on investment—to prioritize your core or new ideas . . . but to use ROI for the experimental investments is really shorthand for 'reduce our innovation.'" Best practice is to prioritize experiments on the basis of strategic criteria or current capabilities. Once feasibility is established, the more traditional financial tools can be applied.

- *Is there one, optimal strategic pyramid?* No. Leadership teams typically develop several alternative strategic pyramids, which should be assessed in the context of the organization's financial position and overall capabilities. Hambrick and Fredrickson (2001) note five key questions that an effective strategy should answer:
    - In which arenas should the organization play? What segments, markets, geographic areas, and so on will be the focus?

- How is winning defined, and how will the organization differentiate itself, and thereby win, in those arenas?
- With what vehicles will the strategy be carried out? Will new capital campaigns, partnerships, acquisitions, and other efforts be needed?
- How are the strategies staged: in other words, what are the timing and speed of initiatives?
- What is the economic logic behind the projects? How will financial targets be achieved, and by when?

Answering these questions is like putting together a jigsaw puzzle. Multiple alternatives of the strategic pyramid and the overall strategic plan are developed. Once a draft set of different yet plausible strategic pyramids is created, the leadership team assesses each from the financial, risk management, and overall capability perspectives to choose what appear to be the optimal investment priorities for the organization going forward.

- *Does the strategic pyramid need separate categories?* As demonstrated by the DuPont example provided earlier, projects should be prioritized in each category. If the wow and core initiatives are thrown together, resources will tend to gravitate toward the most immediate, lower-risk efforts rather than experimental and long-term initiatives. And then, as they say in the Midwest, "You have no seed corn."
- *What if conditions change?* The first question when groups come under financial or competitive pressures should be: "Do we take an equal percentage of resources, people, and so forth from each strategic pyramid category to address the new issue, or do we pluck them from just one or two categories?" Once this decision is made, the "line" separating projects being worked on and those being held in reserve is raised (or lowered if more resources are

available) the requisite amount, enabling organizations to respond flexibly and strategically to changing conditions.

CONCLUSION AND QUESTIONS HEALTHCARE LEADERS AND TEAMS SHOULD ASK

Organizations that manage to blend transformational and current activities are unafraid to change direction and employ clear metrics to determine "go/no go" decisions. No one likes to fail. By their nature, transformational efforts have a higher risk of failure; they must be managed closely to ensure success. Ideally, such initiatives should not be delineated as successes or failures but as learning experiments for proving or disproving hypotheses.

To make such a shift, clear metrics are required for determining whether to continue or halt programs. Such decision-making criteria help senior leaders counter the decision biases that accompany sunk costs ("We are so close. Let's try for another six months given all we've already put into it.") or emotional justifications ("Just think of all the lives we could save if we can find the right formulation."). For example, Google uses the following four criteria to decide whether to continue funding a radically new idea (Goel 2009):

- Popularity with customers
- Ease of attracting Google employees to work on the effort (Google employees are provided approximately one day off per week to focus on topics of interest to them.)
- Propensity to solve a "big enough" problem
- Potential to achieve internal performance targets or objectives and key results

In terms of the strategic pyramid framework, exhibit 2.9 offers a concise strategic plan summary.

The progression in the exhibit clearly articulates priorities and links them to execution, individual responsibilities, and budgets.

Exhibit 2.9: Strategic Priorities: A Medical Device Company Example

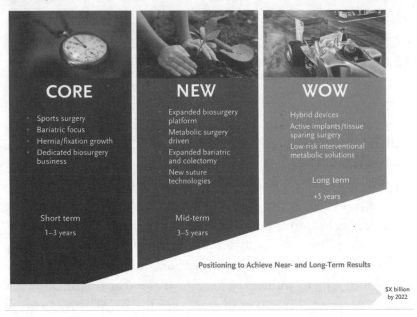

CORE
- Sports surgery
- Bariatric focus
- Hernia/fixation growth
- Dedicated biosurgery business

Short term

1–3 years

NEW
- Expanded biosurgery platform
- Metabolic surgery driven
- Expanded bariatric and colectomy
- New suture technologies

Mid-term

3–5 years

WOW
- Hybrid devices
- Active implants/tissue sparing surgery
- Low-risk interventional metabolic solutions

Long term

+5 years

Positioning to Achieve Near- and Long-Term Results

$X billion by 2022

Source: Adapted from Decision Strategies International. Copyright © 2014.

It is thus both a strategic summary and an operating plan outline that can be regularly updated. In addition, it lists just a few projects rather than the hundreds of ongoing initiatives. Entities struggle operationally when they pursue a strategy of "more is better." As Collins (2009) writes, one of the signs of organizational decline is the "undisciplined pursuit of more." Strategic success and transformative change are built on doing a few things really, really well, not by trying to do everything. As Laura Ramos Hegwer (2015, 18) explains:

> Many healthcare executives aim to transform how their organizations think about delivering care. However, the most successful leaders recognize that what they choose

not to do is just as important as what they actually do during times of change.

Healthcare leaders struggling with how to balance the short-term necessities of keeping current operations functioning with laying the groundwork for future transformational change need to take the following steps:

- Develop a strategic pyramid of short-, medium-, and long-term priority initiatives that can flexibly respond to future uncertainties. Specific priority identification is explored in chapter 3.
- Drive execution with a few clearly defined areas of focus, as covered in chapter 4.

Chapter 2 outlines the rationale for a vision and a strategic pyramid as both the beginning and end of a robust, flexible strategic planning effort for transformative change. To deal with future uncertainty, leaders must first articulate a clear, simple vision for the organization that

- is emotionally compelling, aspirational, and unique;
- establishes the core purpose of the organization; and
- celebrates the values that will be adhered to, even if it hurts.

The vision also sets the guardrails in place for action: what is strategically acceptable, and what is not. The latter is often the more difficult to define. But without that clear sense of the organization's true north and which activities fall outside of the organization's future focus, the trap of "the undisciplined pursuit of more" may be difficult to avoid.

Strategy is about focus. More important, it is about mobilizing all levels of the organization to move as efficiently and expeditiously as possible in the direction outlined by the vision.

The strategic pyramid—the outcome of the strategic planning effort—should accomplish the following goals:

- *Define the short-term, core initiatives critical for immediate success.* Achieving increasingly efficient and high-quality operations must be the goal for all core activities. These functions in turn provide the funding to support the medium- to long-term transformational efforts that will not be revenue or contribution positive in the short term. If the core itself is struggling, institutions have neither the slack nor the resource capacity to do more than survive. However, core investments will not drive transformative change, as, in the words of Dafny and Lee (2016, 84):

  > Simply layering modest incentives to offer services that might reduce costs—care coordination, for example—atop a fee-for-service chassis only results in more volume, even if it is better coordinated.

- *Support a few medium-term, medium-risk new projects that, over time, can expand and potentially transform the core.* In addition, objectively assess where the focus for future efforts should be, and thus where resources and personnel can be redirected for increased impact.
- *Develop a few experimental or wow initiatives that can transform the organization,* accepting that these have relatively low rates of success. The key to managing wow efforts is to "fail fast, fail cheap, and fail often." Learn, reboot, and try again.

Chapter 3 describes how leadership teams can develop a portfolio of options flexible enough to deal with the VUCA world of US healthcare.

Questions

1. Vision
   a. What are the aspirational hopes or goals of the organization?
   b. What would the world lose if the organization ceased to exist?
   c. Why should any stakeholder (internal or external) want to belong?
   d. What are the critical, unique values that the organization supports even if doing so leads to a competitive disadvantage?
2. Strategic pyramid
   a. What are the mission-critical strategic choices in the short-, medium-, and long-term time frames? How is success defined in these periods?
      i. *Core.* What short-term, relatively low-risk investments and strategic initiatives must be undertaken to keep the current organization functioning to meet immediate stakeholder targets? How can core operations be made increasingly efficient to free up resources for investing in transformative (new and wow) initiatives?
      ii. *New.* What medium-term, medium-risk projects have been planned to replenish, and ideally expand, current operations? What initiatives should be eliminated to refocus resources going forward?
      iii. *Transformational.* What wow initiatives could substantially alter the arena in which the organization plays? How will these be managed so that the risk-to-reward ratio of such efforts can be objectively identified and maximized?

Strategy Development for a VUCA World—Scenario Planning

How can you position yourself to win, no matter what the future holds?

—Paul Schoemaker

MANY STRATEGIC PLANNING frameworks are available, as evidenced by a brief look at Bain & Company's Management Tools & Trends surveys (see, e.g., Rigby and Bilodeau 2015). However, as Richard Rumelt (2011) explains in *Good Strategy/Bad Strategy*, most strategic planning efforts produce less-than-optimal strategies. They tend to emphasize generic goals (e.g., "be a market leader," "lower operating costs," "grow market share," "develop centers of excellence in . . .") that lack specific differentiation built on unique capabilities. Some read more like wish lists than strategic plans, with no clear articulation of the operational areas that will or will not be focused on. Such efforts rarely outline a portfolio of choices that optimize current and longer-term opportunities (exhibit 3.1). Worse, such strategic plans do not easily link to budgets, resource allocations, operating metrics, accountabilities, and timetables for action—all critical for execution. As Rumelt (2011, 2) writes:

The core of strategy work is always the same: discovering the critical factors in a situation and designing a way of coordinating and focusing actions to deal with those factors.

Apart from the critical choices that need to be made in any good strategy, which strategic planning frameworks are best suited for addressing the volatile, uncertain, complex, and ambiguous—VUCA—world of US healthcare? Boston Consulting Group (BCG 2015), in an interview with strategy expert Martin Reeves, underscores the point that strategy formulation should be forward looking to reflect current and future realities rather than those of the past:

> Strategy, under relatively stable conditions, has historically relied on concepts of scale, efficiency, and first-order capabilities. But in a world of increased turbulence and unpredictability, leadership is less durable, industry boundaries are blurring, and forecasting has become much harder. We must therefore supplement traditional bases of competitive advantage with dynamic, adaptive capabilities and strategies.

Exhibit 3.1: Four-Step Process: Developing Scenarios

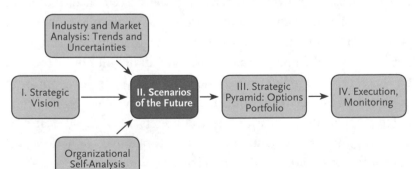

TOOLS USED IN DEVELOPING STRATEGY

Several approaches to crafting organizational strategy are available to leadership teams. This section briefly discusses two common types of analysis and then delves into the main topic of this chapter, scenario planning.

SWOT and Sensitivity Analyses

A favorite strategic planning framework for many teams is a SWOT analysis, which is a template for assessing the strengths, weaknesses, opportunities, and threats of the organization and its possible future environment. While strengths and weaknesses most often focus on the internal capabilities of the organization, opportunities and threats examine the external world.

Once a SWOT analysis is completed, teams typically develop their strategic plan through *sensitivity analyses*, by which they test several variables, such as patient volumes or pricing options, to create estimated future growth paths. As portrayed in exhibit 3.2, sensitivity-derived future growth forecasts are often portrayed as high (or optimistic), medium (or most likely), and low (or pessimistic). (In the author's experience, all future growth estimates are upward sloping; otherwise, they represent a CLM, or career-limiting move.) While the past is not nearly so linear, future estimates typically assume relatively smooth growth trajectories, perhaps indicative of senior leaders' tendency to display overconfidence.

Exhibit 3.3 shows a typical SWOT analysis, in this case for a pharmaceutical company.

Combining a SWOT with sensitivity analyses, the pharmaceutical executive team in this example sought to build on its strengths and mitigate its challenges. While sales appeared to be strong and marketing operations were solid at the time of the analysis, the company faced a declining flow of new, internally researched and

Exhibit 3.2: Sensitivity Analysis

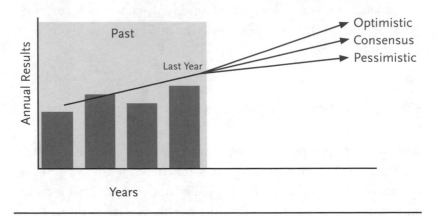

Future Forecasts from Past

Exhibit 3.3: SWOT Analysis

Strengths	Weaknesses
• Strong sales and marketing infrastructure • Ability to drive cost elimination • Industry-leading early-stage R&D pipeline • Robust balance sheet	• Mature portfolio with increasing exposure to generic competition • Lack of blockbuster product launches • Failure of R&D pipeline to deliver on initial commercial expectations
Opportunities	**Threats**
• Movement into high-growth foreign market • Potential to increase sales growth in emerging markets • Strong cash position facilitates potential M&A	• Impact of generic erosion to sales • Development setbacks affecting late-stage R&D pipeline

Note: M&A = merger and acquisition; R&D = research and development

developed (R&D) branded drugs ("Development setbacks affecting late-stage R&D pipeline") during the same period that several existing branded products were coming off patent. As a result, absent any interventions or changes, projections indicated that revenues would decline precipitously in the subsequent several years. To offset these forecasts, the company explored two strategic paths:

- Developing a series of external partnerships with promising, smaller biotechnology laboratories to fill the revenue gap with several new products, leveraging the company's marketing and sales capabilities to drive market penetration of these new, externally sourced products
- Investing in generic manufacturing of the company's branded pharmaceutical products coming off patent

While useful as a quick diagnostic tool, SWOTs are not the best frameworks for rapidly changing, uncertain environments for two reasons. First, SWOTs typically look backward, building off past company and market trends. As explored earlier in the book, in times of uncertainty, the past is not prologue. Second, SWOTs are snapshots in time and thus are often insufficiently dynamic for assessing complex situations because of their overly simplistic portrayals of changing environments.

As for resulting sensitivity analyses, the limiting question is, "Why will the future be any more predictable (shown by linear forecasts) or unidirectional than was the case in the past, especially as future uncertainties increase?" Sensitivity analyses, as well as SWOTs, are best used for short planning periods (e.g., one- to two-year forecasts) or for stable and mature markets.

In the example of the pharmaceutical company, while the two paths assessed were potentially positive, the subsequent discussion quickly focused on only these two. The leadership team missed opportunities for more transformative strategic choices, such as providing its product development and manufacturing processes on

Exhibit 3.4: Choosing the Correct Tools

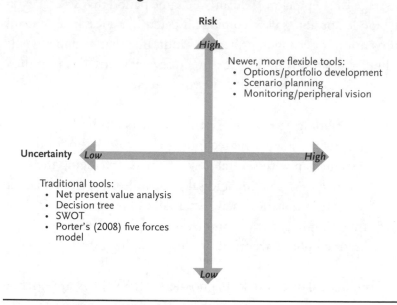

a contract basis to other companies. As articulated in exhibit 3.4, in times of rapid change, new tools and new approaches are required.

Scenario Planning

Scenario planning is the preferred strategic planning tool for dealing with uncertainty. In many planning efforts, options and decisions are developed through a combative mind-set fueled by single-point future estimates, taking the form of "my view versus your view on where we will be in X years." Scenario planning creates an enhanced, dynamic view by allowing the team to "step into" different plausible futures. Rather than projecting from the past, scenario planning *starts in the future* and works back to today, as summarized in exhibit 3.5.

The scenarios are developed to portray a plausible range of alternative futures, as shown by future scenarios A, B, C, and D in the

Exhibit 3.5: Scenario Planning

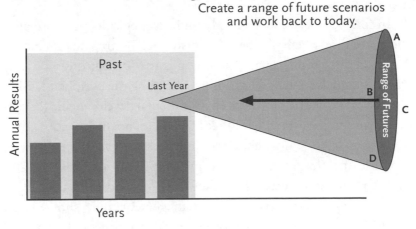

Create a range of future scenarios and work back to today.

exhibit. Each scenario tells a story of how various forces might interact under certain conditions. The key to scenario planning is the ability to step out of today and into different futures. Note that scenarios are not predictions. Rather, their purpose is to help leadership teams generate creative approaches in their efforts to plan for the future. Scenario creation and exploration move teams from combatants to collaborators by pulling leaders out of the present through the exploration of alternative future situations.

Once they are removed from today's constraints and begin to imagine the opportunities and challenges inherent in different futures, senior leaders become very creative. For example, consider the uncertainty surrounding the future of the Affordable Care Act (ACA). Will US lawmakers fundamentally change the ACA? Too many variables are at play to ascertain a sound strategic plan by developing a SWOT analysis and then conduct sensitivity assessments to chart a strategic direction. In scenario planning, however, healthcare teams begin in the future, constructing multiple, plausible futures, such as one in which the ACA is repealed and one in which it is expanded. In contemplating each future scenario, the challenge is to generate a winning strategy, thereby laying the groundwork to succeed *no matter how the future evolves.*

In this way, scenarios not only build strategic dialogue but also, and more fundamentally, help leadership teams prepare for change. A typical output of scenario planning is the identification of early warning signals to incipient change, affording the peripheral vision essential to capitalize on future environmental developments (Schoemaker and van der Heijden 1992; Day and Schoemaker 2005). In a study of 77 large companies, René Rohrbeck and Jan Oliver Schwarz (2013) found that scenario planning helps senior teams improve their abilities to perceive, interpret, and respond to change. Bain & Company, in its survey of top management tools, showed that the utilization of scenario planning increases in times of heightened external complexity and uncertainty (Rigby and Bilodeau 2015), which certainly typifies the VUCA world of US healthcare for the foreseeable future.

Shell Oil's Use of Scenario Planning: Prospering in the 1973–1974 Oil Embargo

While scenario planning has been a staple of military planning since World War II, Shell Oil pioneered its use in the private sector in the 1970s. The company's use of scenarios provides a revealing account of the framework's impact.

At the time, oil was selling for approximately $2 per barrel and most oil companies were vertically integrated, meaning they owned all the parts of their value chain, from the wellhead to refineries to retail gas stations. But several industry experts were worried that the oil industry's stability could be challenged by Iran and Saudi Arabia for internal political reasons.

Led by the company's strategic planning team, Shell created several alternative futures for the global energy market, one of which included an assumption that oil prices would rise to the unheard-of level of $20 per barrel. In considering this future, several points became clear:

- With oil costing that much, the world would likely face economic depression and demand for oil products would be significantly reduced.
- To survive, Shell would have to cut costs dramatically across all areas of its value chain, which executives discussed and prepared for.

When the Arab oil embargo began in 1973 and oil reached $13 per barrel, the company was able to "weather the volatility of the 1970s, bringing financial gains running into the billions of dollars thanks to the re-configuration or sale of refineries and installations, or decisions not to replace them." Shell's moves in this period propelled it from one of the weakest oil producers in the 1960s to an industry leader.

Source: Bentham (2014).

COMMON QUESTIONS ABOUT SCENARIO PLANNING

Before outlining the steps for developing and using scenarios, the following issues are often raised regarding the approach:

- *Which scenario of the future is most likely?* While a natural tendency is to identify *the* scenario to plan for, this approach represents a dangerous diversion. In times of extreme uncertainty, especially in terms of a distant planning horizon, it is highly likely that specific forecasts will be wrong. For example, the primary function of the

International Monetary Fund (IMF) is to aid countries facing macroeconomic challenges by both restoring the struggling country's economy as quickly as possible and containing intercountry economic disruptions. To do so, the IMF projects the future growth of gross domestic product (GDP) on a country-by-country basis. However, as shown in exhibit 3.6, the further out these projections are made, the more likely they are to be wrong.

- *If we do not know which future is most likely, why engage in the process?* First, the purpose of scenario planning is not to forecast, but rather to engage in creative discussions to determine how to succeed no matter what the future brings. Second, scenario planning should reveal, through developing the chain of events that might lead from

Exhibit 3.6: Gross Domestic Product Forecasts Versus Actual Growth: Difficult to Forecast the Future

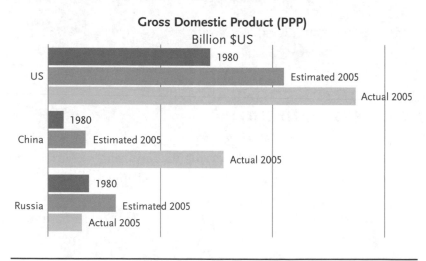

Source: Data from the International Monetary Fund (Van de Putte 2012).
Note: PPP = purchasing power parity.

today to different futures, the critical variables or turning points that teams should watch for as indicative of changing environments. In this way, the organization can proactively—rather than retroactively—respond, as Shell did in thinking through potential major disruptions to their markets (see box on pages 53–54).

- *Aren't there literally millions of potential futures? Which ones should be selected?* The aims of scenario development are (1) to create a manageable number of possible futures to serve as a spectrum of plausible potential futures and (2) to do so in a way that is comprehensible and easy to replicate, not unnecessarily complicated or burdensome. As outlined in the next section, scenario development is designed to spur discussion and open up channels of creativity, not to identify an "exactly right" future to address. It should be a tool to realize a flexible strategic planning process as described by Jack Welch (2005, 166): Strategy is "an approximate course of action that you frequently revisit and redefine, according to shifting market conditions. It is an iterative process."

- *How far into the future should healthcare leaders look when building scenarios? And how broad should their scope be?* Envisioning too far out leaves leaders vulnerable to the risk that everything could change. On the other hand, developing scenarios that are too close in, unless a major upheaval occurs, may be a meaningless exercise, as not much is likely to shift from the world of today. For example, will the ACA change dramatically in the next 12 months? Possibly, but that future is not nearly as likely as the prospect of the ACA changing fundamentally in the next 36 to 48 months. Taking this example a bit further, if healthcare costs continue to rise faster than the growth of GDP—which is their historical path for the past 30 years or more—healthcare spending will crowd out investments in multiple other sectors, from the military to education, which could be a major motivator to change the ACA. What about looking ten years out? That may be too distant a planning horizon, as scientists might have cured cancer by then, for example. Only in the broadest sense do most organizations or groups need to plan for futures that distant.

As to the question of scope, an organization should consider whether the scenarios focus on the national, regional, or local level. Scope depends on the entity and its basic operating environment. A major tertiary care system, such as Kaiser Permanente, is likely to be influenced by macro forces at the national level. On the other hand, an independent subspecialty group of physicians or a single community hospital is more likely to be affected by local or state issues and should focus on factors at those levels in developing its scenarios of the future.

SCENARIO DEVELOPMENT

Building and using scenarios requires three distinct steps:

1. Creating relevant scenarios of the future
2. Using the scenarios to assess the organization's current or ongoing strategic initiatives
3. Reaching agreement on a strategic pyramid or portfolio of strategic investments—short, medium, and long term— to meet both immediate and transformative challenges (introduced in chapter 2)

Each of these major steps involves several components, as described in the following paragraphs.

Step 1: Creating Relevant Scenarios of the Future

Scenario development starts by asking, "What are the critical uncertainties or challenges the organization could face in the foreseeable future?" These are the forces that can change the external environment.

Opposite to uncertainties are trends—those forces whose impact and timing all stakeholders can agree on (e.g., demographic shifts). Trends should be discussed and built into any strategic planning effort. But they are not so-called game changers; it is the uncertainties—*those forces whose timing and impact are not clear*—that can radically upend the world of today. For example, are technological changes a trend or an uncertainty? On the one hand, the onward march of technology may seem to be a trend. However, because reasonable people could argue about the type, timing, and impact of technological change, it should be labeled an uncertainty.

Exhibit 3.7 summarizes factors that should be discussed when developing a list of uncertainties. They are areas that could dramatically change an institution's operating or external environment.

Exhibit 3.7: Areas of Future Uncertainty

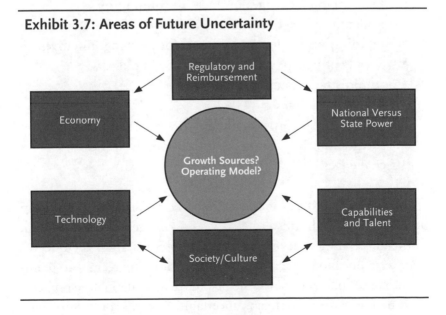

For example, the following is a list of potential high-impact uncertainties that could fundamentally change the future environment for an independent community hospital:

- Reimbursement levels and structure (e.g., fee-for-service, outcomes-based)
- Patient volumes, including by subspecialty
- Competition, today and in the future
- Changes in eligibility requirements for Medicare, Medicaid, or both programs
- Insurance company relationships (e.g., payment cycles, potential discounts)
- Quality indicators and review processes
- Data management systems and requirements (e.g., electronic health record keeping)
- Value of remaining independent versus becoming affiliated with a chain or another system
- Environmental and regulatory requirements
- State of the local economy
- Demographic changes in the local community
- Philanthropic activities and scale of giving
- Funding availability and support for teaching initiatives
- Supply of new physicians, nurses, technologists, administrators, and hospital staff
- Access to capital
- New technologies, including new treatment paradigms
- Integration (horizontal or vertical) opportunities and challenges

The specific, critical uncertainties faced by an organization can be generated by administering surveys asking respondents to rank future uncertainties (developed through interviews) for their degree of uncertainty and impact. More simply, leadership teams can brainstorm a list of uncertainties as the first move in scenario development. Note that with the list of major uncertainties, teams could stop there, forming small working teams to assess the related issue(s) and develop plans for dealing with each uncertainty. (A template for strategic working teams to use for reporting is provided in the appendix at the end of this book.) However, as argued in chapter 1, mental models are hard to overcome. When issues are considered separately rather than systemically, confirmation bias, overconfidence, groupthink, and other decision traps may impede the ability of teams to develop plans. Leaders tend to exhibit more creativity when assessing a holistic future (or scenario) than when discussing each uncertainty separately.

With the list of uncertainties established, leadership teams should move on to choosing the two most interesting or challenging uncertainties with which to create a 2 × 2 scenario matrix (see, e.g., Ringland 1998). Seek two uncertainties that are likely to evolve independently of each other and have a significant impact on the organization's future. No algorithm exists that can determine which two uncertainties are "best." The process involves testing different combinations, searching for the set that creates a reasonable and plausible range of future external environmental factors. One caution is to never choose uncertainties that move together—for example, the direction of the economy and number of jobs, as both of these uncertainties directly influence each other and so respond to other forces in the same direction.

Referring again to the earlier list of uncertainties, the leadership team of a community hospital might choose the economy and the care model. These two uncertainties then form the vertical and horizontal axes, respectively, in exhibit 3.8.

For each of these four possible futures, fill in each future state with a brief description, adding a compelling name that epitomizes that future. Go back to the other uncertainties and consider how each could play out to create the worlds identified. For example, in the upper-right-hand scenario, entitled "All the Young Dudes," the following is a summary of hypothetically "what happened" to move from today into this possible future:

- A growing economy translates into a 20 percent increase in dollars available for hospitals from state and federal

Exhibit 3.8: Example of an External Environment Matrix for a Community Hospital

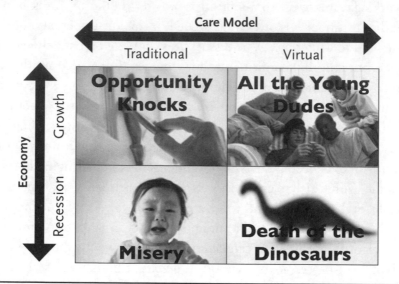

sources. However, continuing certificate-of-need requirements impede hospital expansions.

- The percentage of the population covered by health insurance grows as a result of increased federal support for local insurance marketplaces. Patient volumes at area hospitals dramatically increase, beyond the ability of existing institutions to handle the additional patient volumes.

- Increasingly ineffective antibiotics and vaccines make treating recurring infections, including those associated with the H1N1 (swine flu) virus, more and more difficult.

- Technologies for telemedicine dramatically improve. Major institutions such as the Mayo Clinic and Massachusetts General Hospital handle more patient visits virtually—via video chats, phone consultations, e-mail interactions, and so on—than face-to-face.

- Broadened state acceptance of Medicaid expansion yields experiments in patient management, especially greater utilization of and payment for telemedicine.
- While the economy is growing, federal government expansions of social programs increase the federal deficit. To decrease the deficit, the US Congress reduced budgets for the Centers for Medicare & Medicaid Services (CMS), federal match programs, electronic health record (EHR) system expansions, and in-center medical delivery experimentation.

Is this future likely? The point of the exercise is not to make such a determination. The idea is to develop plausible futures through which to test assumptions about what it will take to succeed in the future. For example, tell a story offering a flow of events that could lead senior leaders from contemplation of today to taking up residence in each of the four futures represented in the 2 × 2 matrix. Be creative; do not worry about exactitude. Just be sure to seek the optimal balance of existing versus transformative strategic moves for success, no matter what the future brings.

Step 2: Assessing Current Strategic Initiatives Against the Future Scenarios

With the scenarios, run a simple test: How well will current strategic efforts fare in each of the different futures? For example, in a world of incremental change, constant political challenges to the ACA, and modestly rising healthcare costs—basically the world of 2017 projected into the future—incremental cost control and EHR expansion will be important for hospitals to pursue. While some growth in the number of accountable care organizations (ACOs) may be seen, widespread acceptance of these models of care is likely to be a long time coming and isolated to a few demonstration projects funded by CMS. On the other hand, is it possible that by 2022, fueled by spikes in healthcare costs and studies "proving" the link between wellness campaigns and declining rates of obesity, more emphasis could be placed on population health? Certainly. Furthermore, in such a future, incremental cost controls will be necessary but insufficient for hospital prosperity.

Exhibit 3.9 illustrates a simple way to evaluate an institution's major initiatives against different scenarios. This type of assessment is typically qualitative. If the initiative performs well in the future, it receives a (+); if it performs as well in the future as it does in the current environment, it receives a (0) or neutral rating; and if it performs worse or does not contribute to the healthcare institution in the future—similar to short-term cost controls in an environment characterized by population health and outcomes-based reimbursement schemes—it receives a (–). The estimated impact outcomes may be color-coded or shaded, as shown in the exhibit, to reveal strengths (areas where an initiative can survive across multiple futures) and to highlight issues (when an initiative might only work in one or two possible futures).

Pursuing an initiative that seems to only work in one or two future scenarios is not necessarily a poor choice. However, be aware of the risks of such an approach. For example, one strategy for retirement account investing is to overweight the portfolio with technology stocks sold on the NASDAQ exchange for their enhanced growth potential. But with that potential comes increased variability and risk as opposed to building a portfolio that combines some NASDAQ stocks with blue chip (established company) stocks and US Treasury bills.

Step 3: Building a Portfolio for the Future

According to a recent study by the Robert Wood Johnson Foundation on possible scenarios for the future of US healthcare, by 2032 the healthcare system could either absorb more than 20 percent of

Exhibit 3.9: Stress Test Example

How attractive is each strategic initiative in *different* scenarios?
(+) = more attractive   (0) = same as today   (–) = less attractive

Strategic Initiatives	Scenario A	Scenario B	Scenario C	Scenario D
Stick to current activities	–	0	+ +	+
Assume risk/ partner around risk	+ +	+ +	– –	–
Network as much as possible	+	+	– –	–

gross national product (GNP) or face sharply reduced spending levels (less than 15 percent of GNP), with the public seeking incrementally "better health" or, more aggressively, "a culture of health" defined by population health and wellness campaigns (IAF 2012). These futures offer radically different opportunities for current healthcare leaders. How can these leaders accommodate both in their planning?

In a rapidly changing, uncertain environment, the ideal strategy is to create a flexible portfolio of initiatives that can pivot, as needed, to meet emerging opportunities and challenges. To do so, teams should identify core, new, and wow initiatives, as discussed in detail in chapter 2.

Next, to move from "stress testing" current initiatives against different scenarios to adopting a specific portfolio of initiatives for the future, break the effort into two parts:

1. Focus on the short term. What critical, core activities will keep the institution functioning—meeting stakeholder needs—over the next 12 to 24 months? If the entity is not producing a surplus currently, the only focus must be on survival. Once ongoing operations yield a positive margin, teams can embark on step 2.

2. Brainstorm a list of new and wow investments from the scenario planning discussions, seeking to identify those initiatives that seem to have high potential in more than one future. Then, perform the due diligence on these ideas to ensure that the organization has sufficient financial, personnel, and organizational capabilities to sustain the investments through the plan period. The portfolio should meet the risk-to-reward profile established as acceptable to the institution (as outlined in chapter 2). Importantly, senior leaders should agree on the metrics for success to apply against each investment to avoid the sunk costs trap.

As noted in chapter 2, the strategic plan comes together when the executive team has reached agreement on a summary that looks like that shown in exhibit 3.10.

Exhibit 3.10: Ranking of Strategic Initiatives

Core	Wow	New
X		1
XY		2
XW		3
SD		4
SX		
SS	A	
	B	
	C	

As emphasized earlier in the book, the number of items is small. Leadership teams should use the 80/20 rule: selecting the 20 percent of projects that will yield 80 percent of the essential future growth or strategic plan impact. It bears repeating that teams encounter problems when they try to accomplish too many objectives. Effective strategy and transformative change are defined in part by the quality of the projects, not the quantity.

The activity itself of listing key strategic initiatives is also critical for execution. Most plans are not realized because they fail in their execution, as is explored more fully in chapter 4. The critical link between strategy and execution is having clearly defined, understandable priorities that all levels of the organization can identify with and manage. Of course, below the high-level summary shown in exhibit 3.10 are multiple portfolios for each operating group that support the overall set of institutional or groupwide priorities.

CONCLUSION AND QUESTIONS HEALTHCARE LEADERS AND TEAMS SHOULD ASK

The only certainty is that the future of the US healthcare system is highly uncertain. Will the ACA be strengthened, fundamentally restructured, or perhaps abandoned? What will be the federal versus state roles for establishing quality indicators and payment reforms? Will a national formulary be adopted, with CMS taking a direct role in establishing national pricing bands for major pharmaceuticals? At what point do increasing patient copayments (often funded through health savings accounts) reduce the amount of care delivered to high-risk populations?

These are a few of the major uncertainties healthcare leaders must grapple with in developing strategic plans for their organization. The challenge is to create, not simply respond to, the future, stepping outside of the tendency to anchor operations in the past. By developing a portfolio of both incremental and transformative initiatives in light of a range of potential futures, healthcare leaders can embrace uncertainty by seeking sustainable competitive advantage no matter what the future brings. To do so, they must

- use the tool of scenario planning to expand their strategic dialogue, thereby challenging current assumptions and identifying previously unforeseen (or unacknowledged) threats and opportunities;
- develop a portfolio of strategic initiatives that can respond flexibly to uncertainties as the future unfolds; and
- focus relentlessly on execution with a few clearly defined priorities, as is examined in chapter 4.

The process of scenario planning enables leaders to view the future broadly, challenging existing mental models and embracing future uncertainties. As Art Kleiner (2003) succinctly summarizes:

> You research present key trends; you determine which are predictable and which are uncertain; you decide which uncertainties are most influential; you base some stories of the future on those uncertainties; you spend some time imaginatively playing out the implications of those stories; and then you use those implications to start all over again and develop a sense of the impending surprises that you cannot ignore.

As discussed at the beginning of this chapter, a key challenge for healthcare leaders is to apply the right tool for their unique environment. SWOT and sensitivity analyses are powerful frameworks that can help teams assess strategic leverage, challenges, and opportunities. However, they are best suited for stable, mature markets that do not typify the US healthcare system in general. For long-term, transformational efforts in times of uncertainty, scenario planning is a more robust, powerful framework.

Questions

1. List future uncertainties/create scenarios. What social, technological, environment, economic, and political (often referred to as STEEP) forces might dramatically change the operating or external environment?
    a. Which uncertainties are most critical? That is, which are most likely to occur and affect the organization?
    b. Are the constructed scenarios plausible and challenging?
2. Challenge existing strategic initiatives. How well will current strategic initiatives perform in different future states?
    a. Is the institution (often unconsciously) planning for success on the basis of only one, or perhaps two, scenarios?
    b. What metrics must be met for the organization to be successful across multiple scenarios, to build in the essential flexibility for success no matter how the future evolves?
    c. What are key stakeholder needs today and in the future?
    d. How might the definition of success change with alternative future scenarios?
3. Create a portfolio of strategic initiatives. What are the most critical strategic investments in the short, medium, and long term?
    a. *Core.* What are the short-term, relatively low-risk strategic initiatives that must be undertaken to keep the current organization functioning to meet key stakeholder requirements? What efficiency efforts will be necessary to release resources for investing in more transformative initiatives (new and wow)?
    b. *New/transformational.* What medium-term, medium-risk projects can replenish, and ideally expand, core

operations? What activities or areas might be reduced or eliminated in the medium term to refocus resources?

c. *Wow/transformational.* What long-term, high-risk—but potentially high-return—strategic initiatives hold promise for future growth? How will these be managed, and what are the clear "stop/go" guidelines to ensure such experiments are neither shortchanged nor wastefully prolonged?

CHAPTER 4

Successful Execution

Well done is better than well said.

—Benjamin Franklin, 1737

STRATEGIES ARE ONLY as good as the results they achieve. And the track record of strategic change in business is unimpressive. John Kotter, in the preface to the book *The Heart of Change*, writes (Kotter and Cohen 2002, ix):

> Examining close to 100 cases, I found that most people did not handle large-scale change well, that they made predictable mistakes, and that they made these mistakes mostly because they had little exposure to highly successful transformations. In a world of increasing turbulence, including unpredictable and terrifying change, the consequences of these errors are very disturbing.

In a more recent study of nearly 8,000 managers across more than 250 companies, the question was asked: "Do you understand how strategic priorities fit together?" (Sull, Homkes, and Sull 2015). The rate of those responding positively was low and varied as a function of the distance of respondents' roles from the senior, strategy-creating level:

- 54 percent of C-suite executives
- 32 percent of direct reports to C-suite executives
- 16 percent of team leaders and frontline supervisors

With such low rates of comprehension, one is not left to wonder why transformative change, especially in large organizations, is difficult to engineer. In healthcare organizations—typified by entrenched hierarchies, complex operations, and highly regulated environments—change is especially difficult.

This chapter outlines the actions healthcare leaders need to take to improve the execution of strategic change (exhibit 4.1). Specifically, they must

- establish a clear *rationale for change* that emotionally engages all stakeholders,
- set *clear priorities* with unambiguous lines of authority and processes for updating as strategic initiatives proceed, and
- create *metrics for success* and steps to take if environments change or results are lacking.

Exhibit 4.1: Four-Step Process: Execution

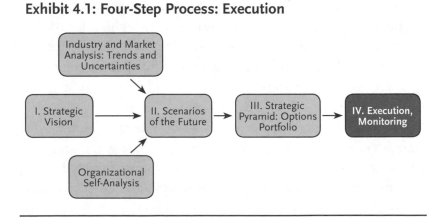

Exhibit 4.2: Common Obstacles to Execution

1. Competitive pressures
2. Conflicting accountabilities
3. Confusion over objectives or expectations
4. Culture not ready for change
5. Unfavorable economic conditions
6. Onerous government regulations
7. Inadequate communication and feedback
8. Lack of adequate resources
9. Lack of follow-through
10. Lack of performance management links to outcomes

Source: AMA and HRI (2016, 72).
Note: No clear statistical difference was found among the items. Span of ranking is 2.80 to 3.06 on a 5-point scale.

None of these actions seems difficult. So, what factors get in the way of accomplishing them? The American Management Association and the Human Resource Institute (2016) studied the major reasons for execution failures and found the issues listed in exhibit 4.2.

From the author's perspective and past experience with numerous change initiatives across large and small healthcare organizations, execution most often fails for the following reasons:

- An unclear sense throughout the organization of "Why we need to change"
- A lack of urgency to change given the daily challenges to meet short-term budget and patient care needs
- An uncertain, sometimes shifting, balance between the established and unchanging true north—the desired future state—of the organization and the need for flexibility to respond to immediate environmental challenges
- Unrealistic time frames for effecting transformative change

All of these issues were confronted and resolved by the leaders at Coastal Medical, a physician-owned, primary care organization in Rhode Island (see the case example on pages 90–91).

The model for effectively executing transformation initiatives is explored in the rest of this chapter and summarized in exhibit 4.3.

RATIONALE FOR CHANGE AND RELATED PRIORITIES

As discussed in chapter 2, the vision for an organization should incorporate aspirational goals plus practical, unique calls to action that move individuals at an emotional level. The rationale for change, then, must be rooted in the organization's vision and should explain "why change" at the individual, emotional level. As Kotter and Cohen (2002, 2) explain, for change to occur, a number of obstacles must be overcome:

> Successful large-scale change is a complex affair. . . . The central challenge . . . is changing people's behavior. . . . Changing behavior is less a matter of giving people analysis to influence their thoughts than helping them to see a truth to influence their feelings. Both thinking and feeling are

Exhibit 4.3: Strategy Execution Process

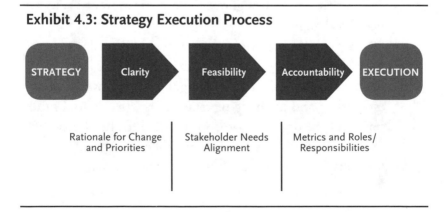

essential and both are found in successful organizations, but the heart of change is in the emotions. The flow of see-feel-change is more powerful than that of analysis-think-change.

The essential and enduring problem is that most people perceive change as a threat. For example, a change in staff responsibilities (e.g., nursing staff being shifted from inpatient care to seeing patients through an accountable care organization [ACO]) usually causes *emotional disruption* for the individual or group. Vineet Nayar (2010a) explains that, in response to any major change initiative, approximately

- 10 percent of the population supports the change (known as early adaptors),
- 80 percent "wait and see" (so-called fence sitters), and
- 10 percent never agree with the change.

What is critical is to sway the 80 percent of fence sitters to support future change efforts by engaging them in each initiative. The keys to doing so are as follows:

- A clear, consistent explanation of the need for change (the "why")
- Clear, consistent messages about the impact of these changes for individuals and groups at an emotional level ("What is in this for me?")
- Clear, consistent statements explaining the benefits of the changes for key stakeholders within and outside the organization

The aspirational vision, developed as part of the strategic planning process, is a major determinant of the value propositions offered by the organization, which employees should hear and internalize during change execution. These value propositions (e.g., enhanced impact on healthcare delivery in local communities) should pull the organization toward desired change. Thus, the propositions should focus on the benefits that will accrue from the strategy and its implementation. Furthermore, they should be explicitly aligned with the organization's overall vision. Throughout the change process, the leadership team must connect emotionally—not just analytically—with all levels of the organization. Slogans are not enough to sway the crucial fence sitters; consistent, personal appeals that guide individuals through the change are essential. (For more on the emotional aspects of change, see Bridges [2004].)

In operational terms, effecting strategic change depends on a clear articulation of priorities. The strategic pyramid, summarized in chapter 2, is the crucial link between strategy and execution. It lists the priorities that must be accomplished for the strategy to be successful. It is the execution "blueprint" for the organization, linking strategy and operations. Ideally, the leadership team conveys the importance of its strategic pyramid throughout the entity and disseminates its content using clear messaging. With this process, each organizational layer is able to develop its own strategic pyramid, which summarizes departmental priorities as well as those initiatives that link back to overall corporate goals.

ALIGNMENT WITH STAKEHOLDER NEEDS

Not all stakeholders are equal. In most healthcare organizations, certain subspecialists are typically granted higher status than other care providers. Similarly, physicians outrank registered nurses, nurses enjoy higher status than technologists, and so on. The question to consider here is: "Will the existing (implicit) hierarchy optimize the transformative changes desired?" As the box discussing the changes at the Cleveland Clinic (see pages 77–78) demonstrates, CEO Toby Cosgrove's fundamental organizational changes in 2008 were aimed at improving care through a patient-centered approach. Outcomes improved and costs were lowered, but the changes were not accepted by all. The Cleveland Clinic's successful transformative change depended on the following factors:

- A strong, well-respected C-suite executive who was willing to challenge prevailing norms
- A successful integration pilot run by a creative, independent neuroradiologist—a subspecialty typically lower in status than the surgeons being asked to join the transformational team
- Board-level support for major, rather than incremental, changes in the pursuit of radically better healthcare delivery

The Cleveland Clinic: Breaking Down Silos

Hospitals are commonly organized into departments by physician subspecialties: orthopedics, obstetrics/gynecology, oncology, and so on. This operating structure reflects physician training and functional expertise, not necessarily operational efficiencies or patient perspectives. Rarely do patients enter a facility requesting an orthopedic consult, for example; they want immediate help for a twisted ankle or a painful knee injury.

As explained by Toby Cosgrove, MD, CEO of Cleveland Clinic, "There is a whole guild system that defines who doctors are, and that guild system is very strong." In the past, such specialization was seen as critical for success in the complex and difficult operating environments that typify hospitals. However, recent technological changes—electronic health records, team-based care models, telemedicine, among many others—increasingly challenge the efficiency and efficacy of such specialization.

Cleveland Clinic's organizational structure typified many of these issues. For example, it operated five separate departments that performed carotid stents with little sharing

(continued)

(continued from previous page)

of databases or protocols—all in an institution that paid physicians on a compensation basis ostensibly designed to encourage teamwork. Realizing more effort was needed to remove operational silos, Cosgrove implemented two major organizational changes in 2008:

- "All staff would be 'caregivers'—not MDs or RNs—responsible for the holistic health of patients (spiritual, emotional and physical); and,
- Organized the Cleveland Clinic around 27 multidisciplinary centers based on broad ailments or parts of the body (e.g., a Neurological Institute combining the departments of neurology and psychology with neurological surgery and other brain related services)."

Cleveland Clinic was ranked among the top ten hospitals in the United States since *US News & World Report* began its annual evaluations. So what was the impact of these changes? By 2013, Cleveland Clinic not only ranked in the top three positions for technical skill for nearly every medical specialty but also "led the nation in patient satisfaction." And where good comparative data was available relative to its direct competitors, the organization ranked lower than each in terms of cost of medical care.

Source: Information from Tett (2015, chap. 7).

- Emotional, not simply analytic, appeals in uniting the organization around the changes
- The Cleveland Clinic's history of innovative, team-based care delivery

While these attributes were unique to the Cleveland Clinic, the point is that transformative change must take account of key stakeholder needs, aligning them in ways that are tailored to each organization's history, capabilities, and resources. Although "one size does not fit all," two components are critical:

- *Key stakeholder engagement.* Stakeholders need to be engaged on the bases of their level of interest and power.
- *Align the organization.* While teams or functions may feel they are aligned to the strategy, rarely is there horizontal alignment across functions or groups to the overall strategy.

On the first point, stakeholder engagement, exhibit 4.4 shows one way to segment stakeholders within and outside the organization to prioritize areas of focus in building support for change.

While clearly most of the time and effort of transformation should be spent working with and understanding the perspectives of the high-power/high-interest stakeholders, effort should also be

Exhibit 4.4: Stakeholder Impact Model

	Low Interest	High Interest
High Power	Keep satisfied and informed.	High engagement.
Low Power	Low maintenance.	Get involved. *Listen.*

expended to manage the expectations of high-power/low-interest stakeholders to avoid surprise concerns voiced by them in decision-making meetings. In addition, manage the time spent with those individuals (often in staff positions) who have relatively little organizational power but wish to be involved in every change-planning activity.

As for alignment, most managers believe their teams are aligned to the strategy but rarely trust that the same is true for other functions. In the Sull, Homkes, and Sull (2015) study of nearly 8,000 managers cited earlier, 84 percent indicated they could rely on their teams to carry out their corporate or divisional strategy. However, a mere 9 percent reported that they feel they can rely on other functions to do the same (see exhibit 4.5).

How can organizations break down silos and encourage broad-based alignment with change goals? According to Brigadier Gerhard Wheeler, CBE (2016), the British commander of the Kabul Security Force in Afghanistan—a multinational force of 1,000 soldiers from the United States, the United Kingdom, Australia, Denmark,

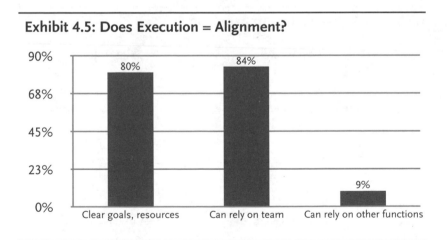

Exhibit 4.5: Does Execution = Alignment?

Source: Adapted from Sull, Homkes, and Sull (2015).

> ## "Man on the Moon": Example of Alignment
>
> In the 1960s, the Soviet Union was widely seen as winning the "space race," being the first nation to put a man in outer space (Yuri Gagarin, in 1961). Shortly thereafter, US President John F. Kennedy made the bold declaration that, by the end of the decade, the United States would be first nation to land a man on the moon. A reporter, between senior administrator interviews at NASA, saw a janitor in the halls and asked, "What is your job here?" The janitor responded, "To put a man on the moon."

and Mongolia—in 2015, the keys to creating unity of purpose and action are to

- understand the issues, constraints, and perspectives prevalent in the environment;
- play to individual and group strengths;
- accept that each group has unique objectives for contributing to the organization and use them to your advantage, as long as they do not conflict with the overall mission and goals;
- avoid creating an "us versus them" environment; and
- show respect, seeking to learn from others.

As Gillian Tett (2015) explains, silos are natural reflections of increasing specialization, data overload, and external complexity. The challenge comes when the silos prevent information exchange or impede organization-wide transformational initiatives. To gain alignment across organizations, Tett suggests the following:

- Keep the "boundaries of teams in big organizations flexible and fluid . . . rotating staff between different departments

. . . creating places and programs where people from different teams can collide and bond."

- Review incentives as "collaborative pay systems, of the sort seen at the Cleveland Clinic. [They] are needed—at least in part—if people are going to think as a group."
- Create a culture that does not hoard information but instead shares data freely, enabling "everyone to interpret information—and let different interpretations be heard." In environments where specialists are prevalent who use highly complex, technical language—as in medicine—the organization may need to employ "cultural translators," who can "move between specialist silos and explain to those sitting inside one department what is happening elsewhere."
- Challenge existing taxonomies and organizational designs, as Cosgrove did at the Cleveland Clinic, to "visualize the world around how the patient experiences health, rather than how a doctor is trained."

One critical question leaders should ask themselves during the execution phase of transformative change is: "Are we able to change course when new information comes to light?" Even Google, with its abundant resources, winnows out innovative ideas using the criteria listed in chapter 2.

COMMUNICATION OF METRICS, ROLES, AND RESPONSIBILITIES

Shell and Moussa (2007), in their book, *The Art of WOO* (where WOO stands for "winning others over"), outline the following keys to successful communication:

1. Survey your situation.
    a. What is distinctive about your issue/idea that you are trying to sell?

     b. Who do you need to be on your side? Why?

     c. What are the communication preferences or biases of different stakeholders?

     d. What will success look like?

2.   Confront the five barriers.

     a. Negative or ambiguous relationships: How to solidify?

     b. Poor credibility: How to develop trust?

     c. Communication mismatches: Does your style fit the audience?

     d. Hostile belief systems: Do you support or challenge existing beliefs?

     e. Conflicting interests: What is really motivating others?

3.   Make your pitch clear, memorable, and personal.

4.   Secure your commitments at the individual and organizational levels.

In the author's experience, communication difficulties typically arise from a lack of active listening and discussion. Many senior leaders—especially strong-minded physician leaders who are trained to make life-and-death clinical decisions—tend to be forceful in promoting their point of view. Successful communication efforts vary from situation to situation, but they typically include the following:

- *Open-door policies/walking the halls.* Leaders should not only be accessible but also seek informal opportunities to answer employees' questions about changes and solicit staff's perspectives on progress and barriers.
    - *Meetings.* For all staff meetings, the execution plan and its progress should be an agenda item. For lunch meetings, senior leaders and stakeholders are afforded the opportunity to engage each other informally on the transformational plan's progress. While often over-scripted and rigidly formal, town hall meetings are critical for broad information exchange. They

also can serve as forums for celebrating milestones reached or updating specific groups on progress made to date.

- *Virtual or physical communication vehicles, such as newsletters and suggestion boxes.* When HCL Technologies CEO Vineet Nayar (2010b, 3) was in the process of transforming the organization, he instituted a "smart service desk" to manage an

> online system that allows anyone in the organization to lodge a complaint or make a suggestion by opening a ticket. We have a defined process for handling tickets (for instance, a manager has to respond to every ticket), and the employee who opened the ticket determines whether its resolution is satisfactory. Not only does the system help resolve issues, but it effectively puts managers in the service of frontline employees.

During the Raritan Bay Medical Center merger with Meridian Health—creating one of New Jersey's largest healthcare networks—Raritan's CEO sent letters in English and Spanish to all staff homes to "keep them updated on the merger and the rationale behind it" (Hegwer 2015, 18).

- *Surveys.* Pre- and post-change employee surveys are helpful for gauging broad employee sentiments and soliciting specific ideas or feedback through open-ended queries. Those entities that successfully employ surveys ensure confidentiality and are willing to engage in two-way dialogue, no matter what the surveys reveal.

Trust in any leadership team can erode quickly if survey feedback is requested and then not acknowledged or acted on in a timely fashion. Those entities that use survey results to maintain or even increase the level of organizational trust

- share results widely,
- discuss outcomes in small groups to ensure understanding, and
- use the findings as a basis for future actions.

For a cautionary tale of the pitfalls inherent in survey myopia, see Fournier's (2001) Harvard Business School case study, *Introducing New Coke*.

The aim is to foster two-way communication, enabling senior leaders to gain a "pulse" on progress and employees to be better informed about—and, ideally, more emotionally engaged in—the overall effort. Successful two-way communication is based on trust. The keys to building individual trust are simple:

- *Competency.* Does the person have the requisite capabilities, or "brain power," to do the job?
- *Reliability.* Does the person meet his or her commitments? For example, if senior leaders say, "We are all equal," but continue to park in preferred spaces or eat in the cafeteria that serves only senior executives, trust is quickly eroded.
- *Emotional commitment.* All levels of the organization want to know whether their best interests are being taken into account at the most senior levels. Does their boss care about their career opportunities, or only how he or she can advance?

Organizational trust is more nebulous but just as important in executing transformational change. Specifically, organizational trust is won by those organizations whose leaders do the following (Zak 2017):

- Recognize excellence.
- Induce "challenge stress"—achievable targets tied to clear progress feedback.
- Allow discretion in how employees do their jobs.
- Enable job choices with accountability.
- Share information broadly.
- Support building relationships across groups and functions.
- Facilitate broad personal, not just professional, development.
- Show vulnerability.

For example, on the last point—show vulnerability—leaders may be faced with questions that do not have an immediate answer. They should respond truthfully, ideally asking in return, "What do you suggest?"

Often, a separate team is formed to manage or implement the communications effort or a specific person is made responsible for the communications plan and its execution. However, overall responsibility lies with the leadership team; its members should be accountable for internal and external communication emphasis, content, and ultimate impact.

OVERARCHING LEADERSHIP ROLES AND RESPONSIBILITIES

Few leaders intentionally under-resource key transformational efforts. Nonetheless, change initiatives can be—and are—indirectly undermined in one or more of the following ways:

- *Focus.* One of the clearest ways the leadership team can convey the necessity of key change initiatives is to reduce execution team members' day-to-day commitments so they can focus on key priorities. McChesney, Covey, and Huling (2012, 11) explain:

> If you're currently trying to execute five, ten or even twenty important goals, the truth is that your team can't focus [making] success almost impossible. This is especially problematic when there are too many goals at the highest levels of the organization, all of which eventually cascade into dozens and ultimately hundreds of goals as they work their way down throughout the organization, creating a web of complexity.

Illinois Tool Works, known for its execution-oriented culture, employs what it calls the 80/20 rule to determine what 20 percent of one's activities are likely to be responsible for 80 percent of results. While qualitative, this rule is an effective guide for leaders to prioritize, and thus focus, their team's execution efforts.

- *Time required.* Often, two related issues are involved in establishing time frames for effecting change. First, as discussed in chapter 1, is the problem of overconfidence. Specifically, as noted by Lovallo and Sibony (2010, emphasis added): "in most organizations, an executive *who projects great confidence* in a plan is more likely to get it approved than one who lays out all the risks and uncertainties surrounding it. *Seldom do we see confidence as a warning sign*—a hint that overconfidence, over-optimism, and other action-oriented biases may be at work." Related to this issue is the (subconscious) tendency to over-optimistically forecast the time required to drive change. Transformative change, especially in large institutions, should be seen as a three- to five-year effort, *assuming focus is sustained.* The question that bedevils many leadership teams is whether the rapidity of external change will be greater than their internal abilities to transform.

- *Ability to adjust.* Every change effort encounters obstacles. The key to overcoming them lies in an organization's ability to adjust. In the case of Coastal Medical (see pages 90–91), the first efforts—decentralizing responsibilities to the medical offices—did not work. So, the leadership team went back to the fundamental rationale for its transformative change efforts, engaging the entire organization and changing course as a result. Observers in the technology industry talk of "design thinking," or the ability to develop multiple prototypes, quickly testing and refining them, and then moving forward (Knapp 2016). To do so, organizations must overcome the sunk-costs mind-set. Gaining objectivity when such decisions present themselves is difficult, but the challenge can be ameliorated by adopting the following recommendations (Hill 2016, 10; Harford 2016, 18):
  - Look forward.
  - Whether one paid $70 or $130 for shares of a popular stock should be irrelevant to one's decision to sell them today for $100. Accept bygone profits and losses as a distraction.
  - Persevere flexibly, not stubbornly. Look for opportunities to redefine the problem.
  - Seek objective outside views.
  - View decisions as experiments that help the leadership team learn. Ask, "What have we learned, and are we still learning?" If you are still learning, the initiative might be worth continuing (if fiscally responsible to do so).
  - Do not ignore negative feedback (beware of confirmation bias).
  - Practice "strategic quitting" by reconciling actual results with the expected outcomes.

Peter Drucker is reported to have argued for "systematic abandonment"—a regular "spring cleaning" of activities or projects to enable the fostering of new business initiatives (Govindarajan and Faber 2016).

Throughout such transformational change efforts, a tension will emerge over whether to adopt a top-down or a bubble-up approach to leading the initiative. In the US military, an officer's job is to articulate "the leader's intent"—the "what" and "why" for any engagement—whereas the troops in the field must determine the means to achieve the intended goal—the "how."

This tension between the responsibilities of the senior leader and those of the "troops" is inherent in execution efforts. One senior executive in communication with the author likened it to flying an airplane:

> Most of the time, I should be at 50,000 feet, establishing the overall direction and guidelines for action by my reports, my teams. But every now and then, I need to be able to drop right down to ground level if there is an issue. My challenge is one of balance. If I am only at 50,000 feet, I lose contact with the market, with the real challenges facing my teams. If I am constantly at ground level, I am by definition micro-managing and no one wants to work for me.

Richard Bohmer (2016), in an issue of the *New England Journal of Medicine*, outlined the following "team-based" redesign approach for realizing major change in healthcare organizations:

- Make small-scale changes to structures and processes over long periods. "Major change emerges from aggregation of marginal gains."
- Use clinicians, with broad staff and managerial support. To broaden the leadership capabilities often lacking in physicians, "transformers invest heavily in leadership

Coastal Medical's Journey of Transformation

Coastal Medical is a major primary care provider group in Rhode Island, caring for approximately 120,000 patients in more than 20 medical offices. Run by physicians, it is committed to delivering high-quality, accessible, cost-effective care. In 2012, the entire organization agreed to provide differentiated patient care on the basis of value, not volume. As Meryl Moss (2016), chief operating officer of Coastal, writes: "In essence, Coastal sought to transition the traditional business model away from fee-for-service medicine to value-based reimbursement with the dual aims of meeting a myriad of robust quality measures while reducing the total cost of care."

Over six months, led by Coastal physicians, each office or practice determined the best way to meet the expanded quality metrics inherent in new, shared savings contracts. The results were sobering: Not only was wide variation found among the Coastal practices, but also no practice achieved the top quartile of comparative statistics.

Coastal leadership realized that the engagement of all employees was essential for transformative change. Through several brainstorming sessions in 2013, the "Primary Care Practice of the Future"—emphasizing preventive care over acute interventions—was established. Organizationally, whereas the medical offices wanted total control prior to the change effort, the final plan centralized basic functions, such as phone coverage and appointment scheduling, allowing the offices to focus on the practice of medicine. Importantly, whereas before the offices were independent, now they operated using standardized workflows, common patient handling processes, and structured data capture to support systemwide quality measures. The results were dramatic: By

2014, Coastal was in the top 1 percent of all CMS Medicare Shared Savings Program accountable care organizations in quality. It was able to easily renew its patient-centered medical home status with the National Committee for Quality Assurance as well.

In summary, Coastal Medical's transformation journey was neither quick nor simple. Transformative changes were ultimately successful because of the following factors:

- The change proceeded from a vision of how the medical staff wanted to practice medicine in the future.
- Leadership sought to engage the entire organization in defining why it needed to change and how best to realize the vision.
- The executive team was willing to support experimentation and pilot programs, making adjustments when results were lacking.
- All internal stakeholders accepted that transformative changes take time to realize.

Transformation is not easy. Coastal created its change through pilots—not one massive shift but a series of smaller efforts—with the lessons learned and then incorporated broadly. Unsurprisingly, not all employees agreed to the new path forward. Turnover occurred, but the majority remained and participated in the change effort. The impacts were, and continue to be, impressive across multiple dimensions, including quality, efficiency, patient support, and employee satisfaction.

Source: Adapted from Austin, Bentkover, and Chait (2016).

development, usually creating their own leadership programs."

- Support experimentation, as "few redesigns get it 100 percent right the first time. In practice, health care transformation is a long series of local experiments."
- Be measurement and data driven, but "make do with the data available . . . treating design change as a test of concept, rather than implementation of a known answer."
- Rely on a senior group for "establishing teams, setting their priorities, monitoring their progress, addressing institutional barriers to change, and integrating multiple teams' work."
- Ensure that unifying values and norms are in place, as "any model of team based redesign devolves authority and accountability away from top executives."

Can such team-based efforts move an organization from fee-for-service medicine to the uncertain, undefined world of value-based medicine, for example? As discussed early on in the book, transformational change means "major strategic shifts . . . restructurings . . . and culture change" (Kotter and Cohen 2002, ix). In the author's experience, such transformational change requires the leadership team's focus on and commitment to a top-down overall effort supported by identified team-based projects tied to established milestones. Organizational efforts that primarily take the bubble-up approach are unlikely to realize the change essential to fulfilling transformative plans. That being said, efforts that are primarily top-down are just as likely to fail because they do not mobilize the capabilities and support of the entire organization.

Transformational change requires a portfolio of strategic initiatives—the strategic pyramid—that both maintains current operations (ever more efficiently) and layers on radical or transformational efforts, as discussed in chapter 2. And such efforts are only as good as the measurement systems that track them. Here, the responsible strategic initiative teams should establish necessary operating metrics for success. As McChesney, Covey, and Huling (2012, 11; emphasis added) argue:

> The kind of scorecard that will drive the highest levels of engagement with your team will be one that is designed solely for (and often by) the players. This players' scorecard is quite different from the complex coach's scorecard that leaders love to create. It must be simple, so simple that *members of the team can determine instantly if they are winning or losing.*

While monitoring change efforts is critical, what if the world changes in ways not envisioned? Day and Schoemaker (2005, 139) challenge senior leaders to be vigilant and open to "disconfirming data":

> What important signals are you rationalizing away? Nearly all surprises have visible antecedents. However, people have a powerful tendency to ignore warning signals that contradict their preconceptions.

Not only should the leadership team periodically review progress against the plan, but it should also spend time considering how the world has changed since it developed the strategy. What new challenges or opportunities are senior leaders *not* seeing? While the warning signs of incipient change in the US healthcare system may be evident, as indicated in exhibit 4.6, too often, industry leaders are unable to "connect the dots."

CONCLUSION AND QUESTIONS HEALTHCARE LEADERS AND TEAMS SHOULD ASK

US President Woodrow Wilson is noted as saying: "If you want to create enemies, try to change something." Change is difficult

Exhibit 4.6: Examples of Market Leaders Missing Embryonic Opportunities

Firm	Market Missed
Coke, Pepsi	Diet/caffeine-free soft drinks
NCR	Electronic cash registers
Keds, Converse	Running shoes
Kendall	Disposable diapers
IBM	Mini- and microcomputers
Friden, SCM, Monroe	Electronic calculators
Anheuser-Busch	Light beers
United Airlines, UPS	Overnight package delivery
Swiss watchmakers	Digital watches
Levi Strauss	Designer jeans
Nokia	Smartphones
Kodak	Digital cameras
Palm (BlackBerry)	iPhone

emotionally, and it enjoys relatively low levels of success in established organizations. Implementing a plan for transformation—the focus of this book—is especially difficult, requiring an aspirational vision, a solid plan, committed management, engaged employees, and dedicated implementation infrastructure.

Successful change initiatives, according to Mario Moussa (2015), are built on the "STAR model":

- *Get specific.* Set realistic, discrete goals.
- *Take small steps.* Break projects down into specific, achievable actions. Once one set is accomplished, move to the next set of actions in a continuous advance toward the overall goal.
- *Alter the environment.* Change the workplace environment and incentives to enable staff to focus on the plan.

- *Be a realistic optimist.* Be ready with a plan for overcoming the inevitable roadblocks to change. And while focused on aspirational goals, be thankful for the small victories that, over time, will lead to transformative change.

Although this chapter emphasizes the steps for successful execution, just as important is an assessment of the organization's "execution readiness." Professor Joe Ryan, who teaches strategy at the Wharton School, University of Pennsylvania, developed a one-page survey for teams to qualitatively evaluate their current capabilities to drive execution (see exhibit 4.7).

Preparing for execution readiness does not mean having all the right answers. The aim is to drive change, thereby moving the organization forward. For as Cato, the Roman historian, wrote (Tichy and Bennis 2007, 14):

When Cicero spoke, people marveled.
When Caesar spoke, people marched.

Ultimately, effective transformative change depends on leaders helping their organization march into a new future for US healthcare.

Developing a strategy for the VUCA world of US healthcare is not easy. Furthermore, strategies stand or fall on their execution. It is not what leaders say but what they do that determines success or failure. To navigate the daunting challenges inherent in strategy execution, leadership teams should start by discussing the questions that follow.

Questions

1. Are the leadership team and the organization execution ready? Using exhibit 4.7, assess the following:
   a. Is the leadership team agreed on the "what" and "why" for transformative change?

Exhibit 4.7: Six Accelerators for Strategic Execution

	Where Are You?
1. Aspirations: • Clear and concise view of the "why" and "what" of the strategy and its implications to my group or function	1 2 3 4 5 6 7
2. Targets and goals: • Translation of aspirations into calls for action	1 2 3 4 5 6 7
3. Organizational structure (macro): • Decisions made quickly with a "bias" for action	1 2 3 4 5 6 7
4. Organizational processes (micro): • The right people in the right positions • Clear goals established	1 2 3 4 5 6 7
5. Performance/benchmark information to assess our progress	1 2 3 4 5 6 7
6. Consequence management • Clear success or failure metrics; timetables in place • Actions taken on the basis of these metrics	1 2 3 4 5 6 7

Source: Personal communication with Joe Ryan, professor, Wharton School, University of Pennsylvania.

> b. Has a clear call to action been transmitted across the organization? To what extent is a sense of urgency evident?
>
> c. At the macro level, is a bias for action present?
>
> d. At the micro level, are staff capable to carry out the change efforts?
>
> e. Have clear metrics for success been established?
>
> f. Will all levels of the organization hold themselves accountable for results?

2. Do the vision and strategic priorities guide all employees at an emotional level?
    a. Is the relationship between the roles of the executive team and the execution project teams clear and equitable?
    b. Are the major strategic priorities clear? More important, do all levels of the organization understand why these priorities are essential?
    c. Are other priorities or responsibilities reduced or eliminated so the organization can focus on the critical strategic initiatives going forward?
    d. Is an ongoing clarity of focus prevalent, or are other priorities being added, diluting the overall strategic direction?
3. Can the plan evolve?
    a. What is the process for updating transformational change initiatives? Does every leader understand the process for updating priorities given changing environments, capabilities, and results?
    b. How will the leadership team overcome the sunk-costs mind-set if changes need to be made in the future?
4. Are the scoreboards or metrics of success unambiguous?
    a. What are the team-developed metrics that enable all team members to know progress to date? Are these metrics benchmarked against best-in-class organizations?
    b. How often are metrics updated? What happens if metrics are not met, or are exceeded?
    c. What are the institution-wide metrics that align functions?
    d. What is the process for cutting back on, increasing, or killing projects based on results? Once projects are under way, can resources be shifted from programs not meeting their targets to higher-impact areas? What are the criteria for making such shifts?

5. Is a viable communications plan in place that supports the vision and progress to milestones?
   a. Are a variety of channels (virtual as well as paper-based, presented at town hall meetings, etc.) being used to articulate common, consistent messages?
   b. Is the content honest, reinforcing core values and key priorities, or is it generic and politically expedient?
   c. Is the senior team emphasizing the same goals and transformative priorities in all their meetings? How will these priorities prevail if budgets are under pressure?
   d. Are efforts being made to align all levels and functions to the key strategic priorities and execution initiatives?
   e. Are information and resources shared for the overall good of the organization, or are departments or groups hoarding talent and resources to protect their turf?
6. Does the leadership team actively monitor emerging external challenges and opportunities? Is the team relatively secure in its views and positions?
   a. What early warning systems are in place to identify challenges or opportunities on the periphery of current activities?
   b. How are these signals conveyed from the marketplace to the leadership team?
   c. How will real threats or opportunities be separated from "ongoing noise"? Who will connect the dots to identify major challenges and opportunities in the future?

Epilogue

When all is said and done, more is said than done.

—Lou Holtz

My dad became a doctor because, as he said, he cared about his patients. He was the first in his family to finish college, much less take an advanced degree. But his family always cared about others. His dad started a cleaning products company in Mars, Pennsylvania, which employed many in the surrounding rural communities. During one winter, when snow closed down the town, my uncles went door-to-door bringing food and water to those in need. The company did well, and it continues to operate to this day.

In these times of mega-mergers and national debates about the costs of healthcare, it is easy to lose sight of the moral dimensions to healthcare. At its core, it is about helping others.

Of course, without money—whether profits for owned entities or revenues for not-for-profits—there is no mission. Yet, the provision of healthcare—helping others—is a social good. This book was written to provide healthcare leaders with tools and frameworks to navigate the VUCA—volatile, uncertain, complex, and ambiguous—world of the US healthcare system. It is meant to help leadership teams transform their organizations to offer more care to more people. For amid all the noise about insurance markets, individual mandates, and affordable care lies the fundamental question: "How can each and every healthcare organization best provide care today and in the future?"

Jon LePook, CBS medical correspondent and professor of medicine at New York University, in addressing the first graduating class of Quinnipiac University's Frank H. Netter MD School of Medicine, advised graduates that managing the "emotional wall" between themselves and their future patients will be challenging (Yale University 2017, 88):

> You don't want to make [the wall] too thin and porous because that can be emotionally devastating. But you don't want to make it too thick and impervious, because then you miss out on all the good stuff, the precious moments when you connect with a patient as a human being. . . . What's going to distinguish you as true healers is the way you embrace humility, compassion and empathy.

When all is said and done, the ability to "embrace humility, compassion and empathy" in providing care for others should be the ultimate measure of success.

Appendix

OPERATIONAL CONSIDERATIONS AND REPORT TEMPLATE FOR STRATEGIC WORKING TEAMS

Typically, several working teams are created by senior leadership to identify and assess potential strategic opportunities and challenges. Three questions that often arise in such efforts are the following.

What is our philosophy of transformation? The overall approach to or philosophy for transformational strategic planning should be one of appreciative inquiry, without necessarily following the available appreciative inquiry models (see, e.g., Cooperrider, Whitney, and Stavros 2008). The fundamental idea is to focus on being positive about future opportunities. All presentations and discussions should support respectful idea generation and exploration rather than participants "selling" their ideas to the group. As Lafley and Martin (2013, 136) explain, strategic review meetings should be dedicated to "clearly articulating your own ideas, sharing the data and reasoning behind them, while genuinely inquiring into the thoughts and reasoning of your peers." However, strong-minded leaders tend to become attached to their ideas and often are uncomfortable when concerns about or potential objections to their recommendations are raised. Ideally, those involved in generating future scenarios come to "live in" the different futures, and as they do, they demonstrate increased creativity and willingness to engage in strategic dialogue.

What should our team look like? Should strategic planning teams be cross-departmental or divided by subspecialty, for example? It depends. If a hospital or healthcare center is raising challenges to current organizational structures, dividing teams by existing structures will be counterproductive. However, if major patient or market segments are clearly different (e.g., elder care versus pediatrics), organizing strategic working teams by those segments or areas of focus makes sense.

If teams are organized departmentally or along traditional silos, an aggregation process will be needed to prioritize the strategic initiatives—core, new, and wow—that are generated across the entire organization. No matter how the teams are structured, they should include a variety of stakeholders to incorporate multiple perspectives.

What is the ideal cadence or pacing for the plan? A typical timeline for developing a transformational plan is as follows:

1. *A kickoff meeting to discuss the purpose, overall direction, and expectations for the planning effort.* In this session, leaders might review or update the institution's vision and develop the first draft of future scenarios. This first meeting can take up to 1.5 days to complete. One key output from this meeting needs to be the rationale for change—the driving vision for strategic action. For some groups, such direction setting is best led by a small executive team. For others, as was the case with Coastal Medical (see pages 90–91 for the case study), engaging the entire organization, though unwieldy, enables differing points of view to surface and produces increased support for strategic change. And without such consensus, driving transformational change is nearly impossible.

2. *Formation of working teams by major strategic area of focus* (e.g., outpatient, inpatient major services, population health). The teams are tasked with developing draft strategic pyramid (core, new, and wow) investments by taking the following steps:

a. "Live in" each of the developed scenarios. Discuss *where to play* (what segments or stakeholders are critical) and *how to win* (what the winning formula for success is)—for each scenario.

b. Aggregate these scenarios to develop an overall set of strategic choices. Typically, the core is made up of those initiatives that will be critical in the short term in the existing environment (or the future scenario that is closest to the environment of today), while the new and wow ideas will allow more flexibility to be successful in different or evolving futures.

c. Develop qualitative responses to the template shown in exhibit A.1. Although this template should be tailored to different situations, the various teams need to use common frameworks so that different team summaries can be uniformly discussed and then combined for an overall assessment of institution-wide strategic choices. Often, developing financial forecasts from the choices made in the strategic pyramid can be challenging. This task can be made manageable by

---

Exhibit A.1: Working Team Template

Vision	Goals	Strategy
Aspirational	Financial: _____	Where to play?
Practical, daily call to action	Reputational: _____	How to win?
Example:	Talent: _____	*Measures:*
Sony: We will change the global perception of Japanese products being poor quality.	Market focus: _____	Quality?
	Partnerships: _____	External rankings?
	Funding sources: _____	Patient satisfaction?
	New program offerings: _____	Community relations?
	Other: _____	Financial ratios?
	Value proposition: _____	Partnerships?
	_____	Other?

approaching it as a qualitative, "order of magnitude" effort rather than employing detailed financial reporting computations. Opt for broad financial ratios, such as breakeven analysis or aggregate revenue/cost forecasts. (The creation of detailed estimates that can link back to budgets follows the second strategic plan meeting, discussed next.)

3.   *The second strategic plan meeting.* This meeting should occur roughly six to eight weeks after the kickoff meeting to allow sufficient time for the working teams to form and develop ideas for initiatives. The goal of the second strategic plan meeting is to review and discuss the outputs (core, new, and wow initiatives) from each working team and answer the questions or topics developed in the working team template (exhibit A.1). Using appreciative inquiry techniques, this meeting provides an opportunity for understanding and challenging ideas and for ideally reaching consensus on choices.

4.   *Aggregation of working team recommendations.* While further detailed work will likely be necessary depending on the questions raised, the effort shifts to aggregating the recommendations of the working teams. This step may take an additional six to eight weeks, especially if specific financial forecasts are required. The compiled and indexed recommendations take the form of a draft plan for the institution, and stakeholder groups are consulted to gain their support and input. But how do teams assess alternatives? The aim is to fit different options together, like a jigsaw puzzle, to achieve a future growth trajectory. Two components are necessary for this type of assessment:

  a. Teams must have a common format for submitting investment initiatives (see exhibits A.2 and A.3). While these assessments might be configured to meet specific institutional requirements, the idea is to have

Exhibit A.2: Strategic Investment Summary Template

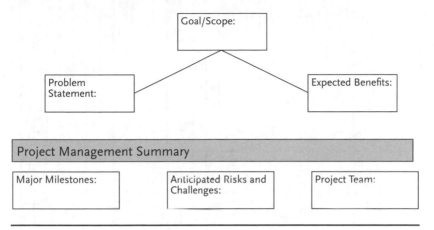

Goal/Scope:

Problem Statement:

Expected Benefits:

Project Management Summary

Major Milestones:

Anticipated Risks and Challenges:

Project Team:

a common submission that will allow comparisons across different initiatives. For example, how might a group compare a suggestion to adopt new marketing initiatives against a recommendation to add customer-facing support personnel? Right from the outset of this consideration, the critical need is to present the suggestions in a common assessment framework that covers strategic initiative risks, investment levels, and estimated future contributions for each.

b. The senior leadership team must base its decision on the organization's or group's vision. Particularly when the alternatives are equally appealing, this decision making depends on the "lens" through which the institution is viewing the recommendations. For example, if the senior team primarily wants to emphasize financial results, the prioritization process will be influenced by this monetary or fiscal lens. Conversely, if the orientation or lens is trained on community benefit—without sacrificing financial stability—another choice may stand out as more appealing.

Exhibit A.3: Strategic Initiative—Detailed Assessments

			Year 1	Year 2	Year 3	Year 4	Year 5	Ongoing?	Total
1. Options for the future (describe actions)									
		Aggressive							
		Realistic							
		Minimal							
2. Incremental investments									
	Financial								
		Aggressive							
		Realistic							
		Minimal							
	People								
		Aggressive							
		Realistic							
		Minimal							
	Other (describe)								
		Aggressive							
		Realistic							
		Minimal							
3. Financial returns or impacts									
		Aggressive							
		Realistic							
		Minimal							
4. Other nonfinancial success metric (describe)									
		Aggressive							
		Realistic							
		Minimal							

CONCLUSION

This appendix offers a generic outline that must be adjusted to reflect the scope and scale of the specific strategic effort being undertaken. Avoid producing high-level goals only; at the same time, do not fall into "excess specificity" such that creativity drains from the organization. Agree on a direction; begin experimenting—while delivering, ever more efficiently, on current operations—assess; and move forward. In this way, organizations can embrace uncertainty through transformational change.

References

American Management Association (AMA) and Human Resource Institute (HRI). 2016. *Keys to Strategy Execution: A Global Study of Current Trends and Future Possibilities 2006–2016.* New York: AMA.

Ariely, D. 2008. *Predictably Irrational: The Hidden Forces That Shape Our Decisions.* Toronto: HarperCollins Canada.

Asch, S. E. 1955. "Opinions and Social Pressure." *Scientific American* 193 (5): 31–35.

Austin, J., J. Bentkover, and L. Chait (eds.). 2016. *Leading Strategic Change in an Era of Healthcare Transformation.* New York: Springer.

BehindTheHustle.com. 2017. "Apple's Manifesto for Innovation and Success." Accessed November 15. http://behindthehustle .com/2012/12/apples-manifesto-for-innovation-success.

Bennis, W., and R. J. Thomas. 2002. "Crucibles of Leadership." *Harvard Business Review.* Published September. https://hbr.org/2002/09 /crucibles-of-leadership.

Bentham, J. 2014. "The Scenario Approach to Possible Futures for Oil and Natural Gas." *Energy Policy* 64 (January): 87–92.

Bohmer, R. M. J. 2016. "The Hard Work of Health Care Transformation." *New England Journal of Medicine* 375 (8): 709–11.

Boston Consulting Group (BCG). 2015. "Choosing the Right Approach to Strategy: An Interview with Martin Reeves." *BCG Perspectives.* Published June 23. www.bcgperspectives.com/content/interviews /leadership-talent-future-strategy-martin-reeves-choosing-right -approach-strategy.

Bridges, W. 2004. *Transitions: Making Sense of Life's Transitions*. Cambridge, MA: Da Capo Press.

Bryant, A. 2013. "Honeywell's David Cote, on Decisiveness as a 2-Edged Sword." *New York Times*. Published November 2. www.nytimes.com/2013/11/03/business/honeywells-david-cote-on-decisiveness-as-a-2-edged-sword.html.

Christensen, C. M. 2010. "How Will You Measure Your Life?" *Harvard Business Review*. Published July–August. https://hbr.org/2010/07/how-will-you-measure-your-life.

Cialdini, R. B. 2006. *Influence: Science and Practice*, 5th ed. New York: Harper Business.

Clear, J. 2017. "The One Word That Drives Senseless and Irrational Habits." Accessed November 7. http://jamesclear.com/copy-machine-study.

Coley, S. 2009. "Enduring Ideas: The Three Horizons for Growth." *McKinsey Quarterly*. Published December. www.mckinsey.com/business-functions/strategy-and-corporate-finance/our-insights/enduring-ideas-the-three-horizons-of-growth.

Collins, J. 2009. *How the Mighty Fall: And Why Some Companies Never Give In*. New York: HarperCollins.

———. 2001. "Vision Framework: Core Ideology Breakout Session." Accessed November 15, 2017. www.jimcollins.com/tools/vision-framework.pdf.

Collins, J., and J. I. Porras. 1996. "Building Your Company's Vision." *Harvard Business Review*. Published September–October. https://hbr.org/1996/09/building-your-companys-vision.

Cooperrider, D. L., D. Whitney, and J. M. Stavros. 2008. *The Appreciative Inquiry Handbook: For Leaders of Change*, 2nd ed. Oakland, CA: Berrett-Koehler.

Dafny, L. S., and T. H. Lee. 2016. "Health Care Needs Real Competition." *Harvard Business Review*. Published December. https://hbr.org/2016/12/health-care-needs-real-competition.

Day, G. S., and P. J. H. Schoemaker. 2005. "Scanning the Periphery." *Harvard Business Review*. Published November. https://hbr.org/2005/11/scanning-the-periphery.

de Jong, R.-J. 2015. *Anticipate: The Art of Leading by Looking Ahead*. New York: AMACOM.

Dobelli, R. 2013. *The Art of Thinking Clearly*. New York: Harper.

Eisenhardt, K. M., J. L. Kahwajy, and L. J. Bourgeois III. 1997. "How Management Teams Can Have a Good Fight." *Harvard Business Review*. Published July–August. https://hbr.org/1997/07/how-management-teams-can-have-a-good-fight.

Evans, M. 2016. "Hospital Firm Retreats as Insurer." *Wall Street Journal*, December 16, B3.

Festinger, L. 1957. *A Theory of Cognitive Dissonance*. Stanford, CA: Stanford University Press.

Fournier, S. 2001. *Introducing New Coke*. Case study 9-500-067. Boston: Harvard Business School Publishing.

Goel, V. 2009. "How Google Decides to Pull the Plug." *New York Times*. Published February 14. www.nytimes.com/2009/02/15/business/15ping.html.

Govindarajan, V. 2016. *The Three-Box Solution: A Strategy for Leading Innovation*. Boston: Harvard Business Publishing.

Govindarajan, V., and H. Faber. 2016. "How Companies Escape the Traps of the Past." *Harvard Business Review*. Published April 26. https://hbr.org/2016/04/how-companies-escape-the-traps-of-the-past.

Grant, A. 2016. "How to Build a Culture of Originality." *Harvard Business Review*. Published March. https://hbr.org/2016/03/how-to-build-a-culture-of-originality.

Groopman, J. 2007. *How Doctors Think*. Boston: Houghton Mifflin.

Hambrick, D. C., and J. W. Fredrickson. 2001. "Are You Sure You Have a Strategy?" *Academy of Management Perspectives* 15 (4): 48–59.

Harari, Y. 2017. "People Have Limited Knowledge. What's the Remedy? Nobody Knows." *New York Times Book Review*. Published April 18. www.nytimes.com/2017/04/18/books/review/knowledge-illusion-steven-sloman-philip-fernbach.html.

Harford, T. 2017. "What We Got Wrong About Technology." *Financial Times*. Published July 6. www.ft.com/content/32c31874-610b-11e7-8814-0ac7eb84e5fi.

———. 2016. "Not Knowing When to Quit." *Financial Times*, May 7/8, 18.

Hegwer, L. R. 2015. "Leading Change from the C-Suite: Three Leaders Share Their Strategies." *Healthcare Executive* 30 (6): 10–18.

Herzlinger, R. E., R. S. Huckman, and J. Lesser. 2014. *Mayo Clinic: The 2020 Initiative*. Case study 9-615-027. Boston: Harvard Business School Publishing.

Hill, A. 2016. "How and When to Stop the Presses on a Failing Project." *Financial Times*, May 10, 10.

Hook, L. 2017. "Ride Hailing Founder Shows Nice Guys Do Not Always Finish Last." *Financial Times*, July 3, 20.

Institute for Alternative Futures (IAF). 2012. *Health and Health Care in 2032. Report from the RWJF Futures Symposium, June 20–21, 2012*. Published October. www.altfutures.org/pubs/RWJF/IAF -HealthandHealthCare2032.pdf.

Janis, I. L. 1972. *Victims of Groupthink: A Psychological Study of Foreign-Policy Decisions and Fiascoes*. Boston: Houghton Mifflin.

Jørgensen, H. H., L. Owen, and A. Neus. 2008. *Making Change Work*. Published October. www-935.ibm.com/services/us/gbs/bus/pdf /gbe03100-usen-03-making-change-work.pdf.

Kahneman, D. 2011. *Thinking, Fast and Slow*. New York: Farrar, Straus and Giroux.

Kahneman, D., D. Lovallo, and O. Sibony. 2011. "Before You Make That Big Decision . . . ." *Harvard Business Review* 89 (6): 51–60.

Kleiner, A. 2003. "The Man Who Saw the Future." *Strategy & Business*. Published February 12. www.strategy-business.com /article/8220?gko=0d07f.

Knapp, J. 2016. *Sprint: How to Solve Big Problems and Test New Ideas in Five Days*. New York: Simon & Schuster.

Kotter, J. P., and D. S. Cohen. 2002. *The Heart of Change: Real-Life Stories of How People Change Their Organizations*. Boston: Harvard Business Review Press.

Kunen, J. S. 2002. "Enron's Vision (and Values) Thing." *New York Times*. Published January 19. www.nytimes.com/2002/01/19 /opinion/enron-s-vision-and-values-thing.html.

Lafley, A. G., and R. L. Martin. 2013. *Playing to Win: How Strategy Really Works*. Boston: Harvard Business Review Press.

Lewis, M. 2016. *The Undoing Project: A Friendship That Changed Our Minds*. New York: W. W. Norton.

Lohr, S. 2007. "Preaching from the Ballmer Pulpit." *New York Times*. Published January 28. www.nytimes.com/2007/01/28/business /yourmoney/28ballmer.html.

Lovallo, D., and O. Sibony. 2010. "The Case for Behavioral Strategy." *McKinsey Quarterly*. Published March. www.mckinsey.com /business-functions/strategy-and-corporate-finance/our-insights /the-case-for-behavioral-strategy.

Mate, K. S., and J. Rakover. 2016. "4 Steps to Sustaining Improvement in Health Care." *Harvard Business Review*. Published November 9. https://hbr.org/2016/11/4-steps-to-sustaining-improvement-in -health-care.

McChesney, C., S. Covey, and J. Huling. 2012. *The 4 Disciplines of Execution: Achieving Your Wildly Important Goals*. New York: Free Press.

McGrath, R. G. 2012. "How the Growth Outliers Do It." *Harvard Business Review*. Published January–February. https://hbr.org/2012/01 /how-the-growth-outliers-do-it.

Miller, C. C. 2014. "How Social Media Silences Debate." *New York Times*. Published August 26. www.nytimes.com/2014/08/27/upshot /how-social-media-silences-debate.html.

Moss, M. 2016. "Creating Ever Better Ways to Provide Cost-Effective Care for Our Community: The Coastal Medical Journey." In *Leading Strategic Change in an Era of Healthcare Transformation*, edited by J. Austin, J. Bentkover, and L. Chait, 107–18. New York: Springer.

Moussa, M. 2015. "Making Learning Stick: The STAR Model." Presented to Wharton @ Work, Wharton Executive Education Leadership Series, Philadelphia, PA, September.

Nayar, V. 2010a. *Employees First, Customers Second: Turning Conventional Management Upside Down*. Harvard Business Review Press.

———. 2010b. "How I Did It: A Maverick CEO Explains How He Persuaded His Team to Leap into the Future." *Harvard Business*

Review. Published June. https://hbr.org/2010/06/how-i-did-it-a
-maverick-ceo-explains-how-he-persuaded-his-team-to-leap-into
-the-future.

Porter, M. E. 2008. "The Five Competitive Forces That Shape Strategy." *Harvard Business Review*. Published January. https://hbr
.org/2008/01/the-five-competitive-forces-that-shape-strategy.

———. 1996. "What Is Strategy?" *Harvard Business Review*. Published November–December. https://hbr.org/1996/11/what
-is-strategy.

Rigby, D., and B. Bilodeau. 2015. "Management Tools and Trends
2015." Published June 10. www.bain.com/publications/articles
/management-tools-and-trends-2015.aspx.

Ringland, G. 1998. *Scenario Planning: Managing for the Future*. New
York: Wiley.

Rohrbeck, R., and J. O. Schwarz. 2013. "The Value Contribution of
Strategic Foresight: Insights from an Empirical Study on Large
European Companies." *Technological Forecasting and Social Change*
80 (8): 1593–606.

Roquebert, J. A., R. L. Phillips, and P. A. Westfall. 1996. "Markets vs.
Management: What 'Drives' Profitability?" *Strategic Management
Journal* 17 (8): 653–64.

Rumelt, R. P. 2011. *Good Strategy/Bad Strategy: The Difference and Why
It Matters*. New York: Crown Business.

Russo, J. E., and P. J. H. Schoemaker. 2001. *Winning Decisions: Getting
It Right the First Time*. New York: Crown Business.

Salancik, G. R., and J. R. Meindl. 1984. "Corporate Attributions as
Strategic Illusions of Management Control." *Administrative Science
Quarterly* 29: 238–54.

Schoemaker, P. J. H. 2002. *Profiting from Uncertainty: Strategies for
Succeeding No Matter What the Future Brings*. New York: Free
Press.

Schoemaker, P. J. H., and S. Krupp. 2015. "The Anticipatory Leader:
How to See Sooner and Scan Wider." *Harvard Business Review*
93 (5): 40.

Schoemaker, P. J. H., and C. A. J. M. van der Heijden. 1992. "Integrating Scenarios into Strategic Planning at Royal Dutch/Shell." *Planning Review* 20 (3): 41–46.

Shakespeare, W. 2017. *The Tempest*, edited by B. A. Mowat and P. Werstine. Folger Digital Texts. Accessed October 27. www.folger digitaltexts.org/html/Tmp.html.

Shell, G. R., and M. Moussa. 2007. *The Art of WOO: Using Strategic Persuasion to Sell Your Ideas.* New York: Portfolio.

Sull, D., R. Homkes, and C. Sull. 2015. "Why Strategy Execution Unravels—and What to Do About It." *Harvard Business Review.* Published March. https://hbr.org/2015/03/why-strategy -execution-unravelsand-what-to-do-about-it.

Taleb, N. N. 2010. *The Black Swan: The Impact of the Highly Improbable.* New York: Random House.

Tappin, B., L. van der Leer, and R. McKay. 2017. "You're Not Going to Change Your Mind." *New York Times.* Published May 27. www .nytimes.com/2017/05/27/opinion/sunday/youre-not-going-to -change-your-mind.html.

Tetlock, P. E., and D. Gardner. 2015. *Superforecasting: The Art and Science of Prediction.* New York: Broadway.

Tett, G. 2015. *The Silo Effect: The Peril of Expertise and the Promise of Breaking Down Barriers.* New York: Simon & Schuster.

Thaler, R. H., and C. R. Sunstein. 2008. *Nudge: Improving Decisions About Health, Wealth, and Happiness.* New Haven, CT: Yale University Press.

Tichy, N. M., and W. G. Bennis. 2007. *Judgment: How Winning Leaders Make Great Calls.* New York: Penguin.

Tucker, A. L., and A. C. Edmondson. 2003. "Why Hospitals Don't Learn from Failures: Organizational and Psychological Dynamics That Inhibit System Change." *California Management Review* 45 (2): 55–72.

Van de Putte, A. 2012. "Scenario Planning and Decision-Making." IE Business School. Published December. www.mile.org/webinar /presentations/Alexlandarwebinar-ScenarioPlanningandDecision Making.pdf.

Viguerie, P., S. Smit, and M. Baghai. 2008. *The Granularity of Growth: How to Identify the Sources of Growth and Drive Enduring Company Performance*. New York: Wiley.

Washington State Health Care Authority. 2017. "Accountable Communities of Health (ACH)." Accessed October 27. www.hca.wa.gov/about-hca/healthier-washington/accountable-communities-health-ach.

Wedell-Wedellsborg, T. 2017. "Are You Solving the Right Problems?" *Harvard Business Review*. Published January–February. https://hbr.org/2017/01/are-you-solving-the-right-problems.

Welch, J. 2005. *Winning*. New York: Harper Business.

Wheeler, G. 2016. "A 'Band of Brothers' Forged from Many Nations in Kabul." *Financial Times*. Published April 4. www.ft.com/content/1711eb46-f1b8-11e5-9f20-c3a047354386.

Whyte, W. H., Jr. 2012. "Groupthink, (Fortune 1952)." *Fortune*. Republished July 22. http://fortune.com/2012/07/22/groupthink-fortune-1952/.

Yale University. 2017. "Class of 1975 Notes." *Yale Alumni Magazine* (July/August): 88.

Zak, P. J. 2017. "The Neuroscience of Trust." *Harvard Business Review*. Published January–February. https://hbr.org/2017/01/the-neuroscience-of-trust.

Index

Breakeven analysis, 104
Bubble-up approach: to transformational change, 92
Buffett, Warren, 17

Career-limiting move (CLM), 49
Castro, Fidel, 13
Catholic Health Initiatives, 33
Cato, 96
Centers for Medicare & Medicaid Services (CMS): budget reductions and, 63; Medicare Shared Savings Program, 91
Chait, Laurence, 33
Challenge stress: inducing, 86
Change. *See also* Transformative change: ability to adjust and, 88–89; being aware of warning signals and, 93; emotional aspects of, 75–76; large-scale, errors and, 71; overcoming obstacles to clear way for, 74–75; perception of, as a threat, 75; questions healthcare teams should ask about, 96–98; rationale for, and related priorities, 72, *74*, 74–76; STAR model and, 94–95; team-based redesign approach to, 89, 92; time frames for effecting, 87–88
Change initiatives: factors related to undermining of, 86–89
Changing conditions: strategic pyramid and, 40–41
Cialdini, Robert, 25
Clarity: in strategy execution process, *74*
Cleveland Clinic: breaking down silos at, 77–78; incentives as collaborative pay systems at, 82; transformative change at, 76, 77–79; *U.S. News & World Report* ranking for, 78
CLM. *See* Career-limiting move

CMS. *See* Centers for Medicare & Medicaid Services
Coastal Medical (Rhode Island): transformative change at, 74, 88, 90–91, 102
Cognitive errors: safeguarding against, 18
Communication, successful: keys to, 82–83; open-door policies/walking the halls and, 83–84; organizational trust and, 85–86; surveys and, 84–85; two-way, 85; virtual or physical communication vehicles and, 84
Communications plan: questions related to, 98
Compassion: embracing, 100
Competency: trust and, 85
Confirmation bias, 4, 7–10, 61, 88; financial meltdown of 2007–2008 and, 8; offsetting, 14; overconfidence and, 8–9; questions to discuss relative to, 19
Consequence management: strategic execution and, *96*
Core ideas: prioritizing, 39
Core initiatives: flexible portfolio of initiatives and, 65; formation of working teams and, 102; organizational goals and, 44; questions related to, 45, 69; ranking of, 37, *37*; second strategic plan meeting and, 104; strategic priorities: medical device company example, *42*; in strategic pyramid, 31, *31, 32*, 36
Core purpose, 31; in compelling vision, 27–28; examples of, 26–27
Corporate value statements, 28
Cosgrove, Toby, 76, 77, 78, 82
Cote, David M., 3
Covey, Stephen, 21

FrontPoint Partners, 8
Future scenarios: assessing current
    strategic initiatives against, 58,
    63–64

Generic goals, 47
GNP. *See* Gross national product
Goal(s): aspirational, 22, 27; focus
    and, 86–87; generic, 47; realistic,
    discrete, 94; strategic execution
    and, *96*; strategic pyramid and,
    44; of strategies, 33
Good Strategy/Bad Strategy (Rumelt),
    47
Google: criteria for funding radically
    new ideas, 41, 82
Govindarajan, Vijay: box 1/box 2/box
    3 framework of, 31
Grant, Adam, 12
Groopman, Jerome, 18
Gross national product (GNP), 65
Groupthink, 5, 10–15, 61; avoiding
    perils of, 12–15; disrupting, 12;
    JFK and Cuban Missile Crisis
    and, 13; power of, 11; questions
    related to, 19

Harari, Yuval, 12
Healthcare organizations: gaining
    alignment across, 81–82
Healthcare reform: questions to ask
    about, 9–10
Heart of Change, The (Kotter), 71
Hegwer, Laura Ramos, 42
Herbert, David, 34
Hewlett-Packard. *See* HP Develop-
    ment Company
Holtz, Lou, 99
Hospitals: studying organizational
    failures at, 17
How Doctors Think (Groopman), 18
HP Development Company: core
    purpose statement for, 26

Human Resource Institute: on
    common obstacles to execution,
    73, *73*
Humility: embracing, 100

Illinois Tool Works, 87
IMF. *See* International Monetary
    Fund
Incentives: as collaborative pay sys-
    tems, 82
Independent data: avoiding group-
    think and use of, 14
Influence (Cialdini), 25
Initiatives: incremental and trans-
    formative, 67–68. *See also* Core
    initiatives; New initiatives;
    Portfolio of initiatives; Strategic
    initiatives; Wow initiatives
International Monetary Fund (IMF):
    gross domestic product forecasts
    vs. actual growth, 56, *56*
Internet: polarization and, 3
Introducing New Coke (Fournier),
    85

Janis, Irving: on power of group-
    think, 11

Kabul Security Force (Afghanistan),
    80–81
Kahneman, Daniel, 2
Kaiser Permanente, 58
Kennedy, John F.: Cuban Missile
    Crisis and, 13
Kleiner, Art, 68
Kleiner Perkins Caufield & Byers
    (KPCB), 15
Kotter, John, 71

Langer, Ellen, 24, 25
Leaders: all points of view considered
    by, 3; learning from challenges
    and, 16; organizational trust

and, 85–86; questions asked by, 41; questions related to decision traps for, 18–19

Leadership roles and responsibilities: ability to adjust and, 88–89; focus and, 86–87; time frame and, 87–88

LePook, Jon, 100

Listening: active, lack of, 83

Lohr, Steve, 1

Lyft: values statement for, 28

Managed capital, drivers of return on, 9, *10*

"Man on the moon" alignment example, 81

Mary Kay: core purpose statement for, 26

Massachusetts General Hospital, 62

Mayo Clinic, 62; core purpose statement for, 26; 2020 strategic plan, 33–34

McGrath, Rita Gunther: practices of outliers for sustaining growth, *35, 35,* 36

McKinsey & Company: core purpose statement for, 26; "three horizons for growth" concept, 31

Meetings: execution plan and, 83–84; in transformational plan timeline, 102, 104

Merck: core purpose statement for, 26

Meridian Health: merger with Raritan Bay Medical Center, 84

Metrics: consequence management and, *96*; decision-making criteria and, 41; questions related to, 97; scorecards, 93; strategy execution process and, *74*; working team template 61, *103*; for success, creating, 72, 82–86

Mission: vision and, 21–22

Model T automobile: Ford's vision for, 23–24

Morgan Stanley, 8

Moss, Meryl, 90

NASDAQ, 64

National Committee for Quality Assurance, 91

Nayar, Vineet, 75, 84

Negative feedback: awareness of, 88

New England Journal of Medicine, 89

New ideas: prioritizing, 39

New initiatives: brainstorming list of, 66; enabling, systematic abandonment and, 89; flexible portfolio of initiatives and, 65; formation of working teams and, 102; organizational goals and, 44; questions related to, 45, 69–70; ranking of, 37, *37;* second strategic plan meeting and, 104; strategic priorities: medical device company example, *42;* in strategic pyramid, 31, *31,* 32, 36

Newsletters: transformative change and, 84

Nike: core purpose statement for, 26

Objectivity: gaining, 88

Oil embargo of 1973–1974: Shell Oil's use of scenario planning and, 54–55, 57

Open-door policies, 83–84

Optimism: realistic, 95

Organizational decline: signs of, 42

Organizational structure: strategic execution and, *96*

Organizational trust: avoiding groupthink and, 14; winning, 85–86

Organizational values: compelling vision and, 28

Tenet Healthcare, 33
Tett, Gillian, 81
"Three horizons for growth" concept
    (McKinsey & Company), 31
3M: core purpose statement, 26
Time frames: for effecting change,
    87–88; for strategic pyramid,
    38–39
Top-down approach: to transforma-
    tional change, 92
Toyota Production System, 28
Transformational plan, timeline for,
    102–5; aggregation of working
    team recommendations, 104–5;
    formation of working teams,
    102–3; kickoff meeting, 102; sec-
    ond strategic plan meeting, 104
Transformative change: alignment
    with stakeholder needs and,
    76–82; at Cleveland Clinic,
    76, 77–79; at Coastal Medical
    (Rhode Island), 74, 88, 90–91,
    102; defining, 92; difficulty in
    engineering, 72; embracing
    uncertainty through, 107; guided
    by vision, 30–31; hierarchical
    status issues and, 76; initiating,
    24–25; new information and
    changing course in, 82; quality of
    projects and, 67; strategic success
    and, 42–43; time frames for, 73,
    87
Trends: uncertainties vs., 59
Trust. See Organizational trust
Twain, Mark, 1
2 × 2 scenario matrix: creating, 61–62
Two-way communication: fostering,
    85

Uber: values statement for, 28
Uncertainty(ies). See also VUCA (vol-
    atile, uncertain, complex, and
    ambiguous) world: embracing

through transformational
    change, 107; future, areas of, 59,
    59–60; organizational vision and,
    43; potential high-impact, list
    of, 60; questions related to, 69;
    scenario planning and, 52, 68;
    strategic planning and grappling
    with, 67; trends vs., 59; 2 × 2
    scenario matrix and, 61
"Undisciplined pursuit of more" trap:
    challenge in avoiding, 43; organi-
    zational decline and, 42
U.S. News & World Report, 78

Value-based reimbursement model:
    at Coastal Medical, 90–91
Value propositions: aspirational
    vision and, 75–76
Values: in compelling vision, 28; core,
    31
Values statement: employee guidance
    in, 28–29
Video chats, 62
Virginia Mason Health System: on
    "rocks in your shoes" problems,
    32
Vision: aspirational, value proposi-
    tions and, 75–76; clinical subspe-
    cialty example, 30; compelling,
    components of, 27–28; develop-
    ing, 22–29; future uncertainty
    and, 43; mission and, 21–22;
    participants in creating, 29–31;
    priorities and, 22; questions
    related to, 45, 97; rationale for
    change and, 74; revising, 30
Vision statements: creating, 29, 29;
    examples of, 23; intention setting
    and, 22; organizational unique-
    ness and, 24
VUCA (volatile, uncertain, complex,
    and ambiguous) world, 99. See
    also Uncertainty(ies); addressing,

About the Author

Jim Austin, a former senior executive at Baxter Healthcare, combines business strategy and organizational development theory with extensive industry experience to guide organizations and individuals as a consultant and an educator. He spent 12 years at Baxter, the last 4 as vice president of strategy development for the renal division, a rapidly growing, nearly $2 billion business. Before that, Jim was assistant to the president for ANCHOR HMO, a subsidiary of Rush Medical Center in Chicago. Prior to his move to Chicago, he worked as a consultant for Arthur D. Little Inc., where he led a number of large-scale planning, business development, and strategic positioning studies. Between college and graduate school, he spent four years as an economist and a planning officer in the Ministry of Finance of Botswana.

More recently, Jim worked at Decision Strategies International from 2005 to 2016, leaving as a senior principal. There, he led numerous projects, including the development of scenarios of the future for a medical devices firm, research and development priorities for a major consumer products company, a strategic plan for the American College of Radiology, and scenarios of the future for the League of Southeastern Credit Unions. He now heads his own strategy and executive development firm, JH Austin Associates Inc. (www.jh-austin.com).

In 2013, Jim was appointed by Brown University as an adjunct senior lecturer in the Executive Master of Healthcare Leadership program, heading a graduate marketing and management course.

He is a faculty member at Duke Corporate Education, delivering senior-level seminars on strategy, strategic execution, innovation, and decision making for a range of banking, pharmaceutical, and other industry clients. Jim is also a lecturer/consultant at the Aresty Institute of Executive Education in the Wharton School, where he tailors and delivers senior-level seminars for a number of leading companies.

Jim holds a bachelor of arts degree in economics and politics from Yale University. He was a Special Student at the Massachusetts Institute of Technology in the Urban Studies Department, and he received a joint master of public affairs/master of urban and regional planning degree from the Woodrow Wilson School at Princeton University. Previously, Jim was chairman of the Strategic Leadership Forum, a board member of the National Kidney Foundation of Illinois, a member of the board of directors for the University Club of Chicago, treasurer of LaSalle Language Academy, and a member of the admissions committee for the Latin School of Chicago.